GORDON & ALEXA –

TO SUCCESS IN ALL
YOU DO!

x MATT x

Rockon!!

The Boomerang Effect

for Dental Professionals

The Boomerang Effect

for Dental Professionals

How Your Beliefs Return to Create Your Personal and Professional Lives

Dr. Matthew J. Bynum
Dr. Arthur J. Mowery, Jr.

Hakalau Publishing Company
Simpsonville, South Carolina

First printing 2008

ISBN 978-0-9801116-4-4

LCCN 2007940212

ATTENTION CORPORATIONS, UNIVERSITIES, COLLEGES, AND PROFESSIONAL ORGANIZATIONS: Quantity discounts are available on bulk purchases of this book for educational, gift purposes, or as premiums for increasing magazine subscriptions or renewals. Special books or book excerpts can also be created to fit specific needs. For information, please contact Hakalau Publishing Company, 1334 S. Hwy 14, Simpsonville, SC 29681.

Dedication

To our beautiful wives, Ann and Kim, and our adorable children, Matthew, Luke, and John, and Morgan and Jake. Your understanding, patience, and love are appreciated as we pursue our passions of teaching and inspiring others to live their dreams. We love you!

Contents

Section 3: Harmonic Wealth®

Acknowledgments

There are two authors of this book, but there are many people who have aided our journeys in life. Special thanks to Dr. Bill Dickerson and James Arthur Ray, who have been our trusted teachers and mentors for years. We appreciate your wisdom and friendship.

We would also like to acknowledge the team and alumni of the Las Vegas Institute of Advanced Dental Studies (LVI) for supporting our *Achieving Extreme Success* seminar series and coaching programs.

We are forever grateful to the dentists and their teams who have allowed us to teach, coach, and inspire them on their life journeys. We are honored to be with you and thank you for the confidence you've placed in us.

Our fellow instructors at LVI have influenced us tremendously. We appreciate your sharing of clinical, practice management, and life skills ideas.

We would not be where we are today without the very special ladies who work with us in our offices. They make it a joy to walk in the door.

We would like to thank our good friend Nate Booth for helping us transform the ideas in our heads to words on paper. We think you will agree the people at About Books, Inc.

did a fantastic job of making the book easy and enjoyable to read.

Finally, we would like to acknowledge you for reading this book. The topic is very unusual for dentistry, and it says a lot that you chose to explore the topic of beliefs.

Foreword

Have you ever met someone and immediately known that person was destined for greatness? That happened to me in 1998 when I met Matt Bynum and Art Mowery at the Las Vegas Institute for Advanced Dental Studies. They were both in their thirties, but something was very different about them.

Five years later, when I attended one of their early *Achieving Extreme Success* seminars, I discovered what the difference was. At a relatively young age, they had learned that *the important lessons of dentistry are the important lessons of life.* They talked about creating high-performance teams you could trust and practicing dentistry the way *you* think it should be done instead of following what other people and groups think you should do. They talked about learning to love dentistry, your team, and your patients. They talked about dentists needing to loosen up and making the office environment more fun.

At that time, I told them they should write a book about these important lessons. The time wasn't right, so the project never got started. Then in 2007, I attended another *Achieving Extreme Success* seminar. The first one I attended was really good. This one was really great. They enthusiastically communicated what dentists need to do *and* what beliefs they need to hold. I wrote down ten of these empowering beliefs and told them again, "You need to write a book about this stuff!" Luckily, they listened to me this time. The book you have in your hands is the result.

Sometimes in dentistry, in our drive to be proper and professional, we squeeze all the passion and joy out of our communication. Matt and Art want no part of this constriction. They're into expansion—on both professional and personal levels. *The Boomerang Effect for Dental Professionals* will expand your knowledge of the inner workings of your mind and *How Your Beliefs Return to Create Your Personal and Professional Lives.* This book is a bountiful harvest of knowledge that will enable you to create the practice of your dreams. Read it and reap the rewards!

Nate Booth DDS, MS
Author of the books *Tiger Traits; The Diamond Touch; Thriving on Change; Let the Chips Fall Where They May*; and co-author of the books *555 Ways to Reward Your Dental Team; How to Create an Exceptional Aesthetic Practice; Unleashing the Power of Dentistry; Change Your Smile, Change Your Life®*; and *Change Your Bite, Change Your Life*

"The game of life is a game of boomerangs. Our thoughts, deeds, and words return to us sooner or later, with astounding accuracy."

—Florence Shinn

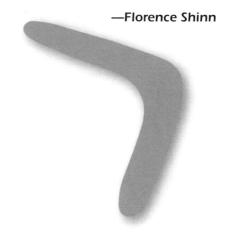

Introduction

There are dozens of books written each year for dentists. In one way or another, they all focus on what you need to *do* to create success. They tell you how to do an exam, diagnose patients, prep teeth, market your practice, design your office, schedule your day, hire and train people, and build wealth. This book is different. It focuses on doing *and* being—not just doing. It focuses on actions *and* beliefs—not just actions.

You might be thinking right now, "Concepts like 'being' and 'beliefs' are the soft stuff that doesn't have a place in the daily challenge of running a dental practice. I've got bills to pay, teeth to cut, and problems to solve."

We're here to tell you that the soft stuff has *everything* to do with your success and happiness. It determines how you think and feel, what you do, and the results you achieve—in dentistry and in life! But here's the kicker—enhancing the soft stuff is the most challenging work you'll ever do. It's easy to change how you prep a tooth. It's challenging to change your beliefs.

We believe a challenge is good for two reasons:

1. Think of anything you truly value in life—your dental degree, successful dental practice, or an important relationship. Was it easy or challenging attaining and maintaining them? For most people it took some time and effort.

2. If transforming beliefs were easy, almost everybody would do it. The fact that it's challenging, and you're willing to do it, gives you the opportunity to create practice separation from everybody else.

Our Journeys

As you will discover in the chapters that follow, the dental practices we've created are direct results of our beliefs. To understand how our beliefs came to be, it's important to be familiar with our journeys through life.

Matt's Journey

As an undergraduate at the University of California at San Diego, I majored in the three "Bs"—baseball, beer, and the beach. My budding baseball career came to a screeching halt when I seriously injured my shoulder playing intramural football. So, with a sparkling 2.7 GPA and roller coaster-like DAT scores, I visited four Midwestern dental schools in five days. I'll never know for sure what the University of Iowa saw in me, but two days after the interview they sent me an acceptance letter.

We Didn't Mess with Texas

My wife, Ann, and I graduated from dental school in 1995. We packed up the Family Truckster and headed south to San Antonio, where Ann did a two-year pediatric residency. While in San Antonio, I was extremely lucky to work for a fine restorative dentist, Dr. Craig Carlson. I learned two very important lessons while working in Craig's practice:

1. The office was what I call *traditional* fee-for-service practice. The patients made partial payment to the office before their care. Then, the office billed the insurance company for the balance. Finally, the office billed the patients

for the balance. As a result, insurance considerations seemed to interfere with providing quality, comprehensive dentistry to my patients. In addition, there were two full-time front desk people who did nothing but deal with the insurance companies. I swore that when I started my own practice it would be *true* fee-for-service, in which patients would pay me in advance for their care, file their own claims with office-generated forms, and then receive reimbursements directly from the insurance companies.

2. I learned from Craig that dentistry is not a tooth and gum business. It's a relationship business. Craig was a master at forming close, new relationships and maintaining existing ones. I saw that the success of his practice was primarily due to the deep and lasting friendships he formed. I've never forgotten that.

Here's an excellent example of the power of relationships. While working in Craig's office, I did my first full-mouth reconstruction case on a man I'll call John. John and his wife, Carol, became very good friends with Ann and me. When we made the decision to start our practice in Simpsonville, South Carolina, he offered to help. His $100,000 unsecured loan paid for the land on which we built our dream office. I took the deed for the land to four banks before the fifth one loaned us the money to construct our six thousand-square-foot, $650,000 building. It would have been extremely difficult for Ann and me to start the way we did without the help of our friends.

Go Big or Go Home

Ann and I wanted to create a true family practice in which adults would be seen by a general dentist with extensive training in restorative dentistry and children would be seen by a pediatric specialist. That way we could create some nice synergies in terms of attracting entire families. We could also cross-refer.

It was important for our building to be a physical representation of the quality dentistry we were going to provide. One of the best marketing ideas I've ever had was to put up a big sign that said "Future Home of Hollytree Family Dental" in front of the building as it was being built. It generated a lot of talk in the community. We even had people drive by the office, hop out of their cars, and walk through the unfinished building. Best of all, our new building began the process of creating practice separation from the other dentists in town. We'll talk more about practice separation in the chapter on Core Belief #4: To Have Different, I Must Do Different.

Great Scott!

In 1998 I made another important decision. I decided to attend the Las Vegas Institute for Advanced Dental Studies (LVI). At the first course, I met a Scotsman by the name of David Philip, who looked like he was in his seventies. During the week, I talked with David a lot. He spoke of his dental journey, which covered more years than I'd been alive! He eloquently praised LVI's teachings, which were precisely in line

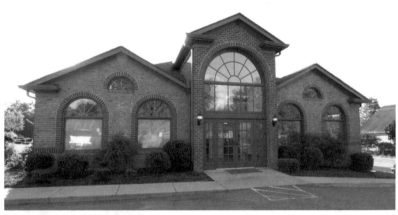

The exterior of Matt's office.

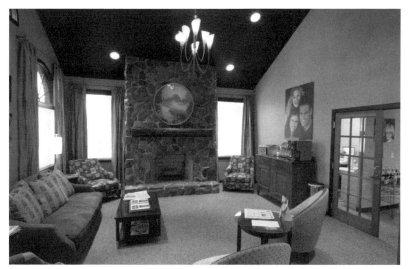

The interior of Matt's office.

with what he believed it took to be successful in dentistry and in life. David spoke from experience. More importantly, he spoke from his heart.

The last day of the program, David stood up in front of the group and gave a short talk I will never forget. He basically told his life story. As a younger man, he was a very successful dentist. He would get busy and add a hygienist and another treatment room. He would get busier and add an assistant or two. He would get even busier and add an associate, more assistants, and more treatment rooms.

David's pattern of continual adding repeated itself for many years. Then, one day, David got a phone call informing him that his son had died in a car accident. If that wasn't bad enough, David had a severe heart attack a few months later.

These two events got David thinking about what was truly important in his life—and being busy at the office wasn't one of them. David decided that being with his family and only doing the types of dentistry he loved were the most important personal and professional goals for him. From that point on, he arranged his life so he could do both. He reduced the number of people on his team. He shortened the time he spent at the office and spent more time with his family. And guess what? He made *more* money.

Hearing David's story was a defining moment for me because, at the time, I was exactly where he was before his son's death. I was adding and adding and adding. I was seeing patients Monday through Thursday for eight hours a day. I didn't get home until at least six o'clock on most nights. On Friday, I saw patients in the morning but did administrative chores in the afternoon. I also worked every other Saturday. In addition to all the time I was spending at the office, my first child, Matthew II, had just been born. I wanted to spend more time with Ann and him.

After listening to David, I chose to change the way I practiced dentistry and lived my life. David gave me the spark to get started, and LVI gave me the clinical and business skills to finish the job. The spark and the skills have definitely produced their desired effect. In 2006 I worked 123 days and grossed around $1.5 million. More importantly, I love what I do. I love the people I do it with. And I love the people I do it for.

David Philip helped me break a paradigm that was holding me back. A paradigm is a theoretical framework that influences a broad area of behavior. Two extremely damaging paradigms that have been systematically taught to dentists for years are "Busy is better" and "When you get busy, you add." Art and I have found the exact opposite to be true. We believe that "Busy is not better" and "When you get busy, you subtract." Later in the book, you will learn how paradigms can create a variety of unwritten rules that limit your professional success and personal happiness.

Art's Journey

I graduated from the University of Florida, College of Dentistry, in 1996. After graduation, I did a one-year general practice residency. A corporation that owned dozens of practices in the Southeast opened an office in Gainesville about the time I finished my residency. I made the decision to work for them. It was great at first! I had forty patients a day walking through the doors to see me. This was my first chance to use my freshly-honed dental skills on real people to save the world.

I was determined to become one of the top-producing dentists in the fifty-office chain. I achieved my goal by working ten to twelve hours a day, five days a week. At the peak of my insanity I was seeing sixty patients a day, routinely running two hours behind schedule, and never stopping for lunch. My production averaged a staggering $2,900 a day.

I huffed and puffed on that treadmill for six months. During that time my enthusiasm for dentistry gradually dwindled. Finally, I couldn't take it anymore. I went home and told my wife, Kim, "I made a mistake becoming a dentist. I think I'll quit my hamster-on-a-wheel job and go pour Slurpees at a 7-Eleven for a while."

As strange as it might seem, I look back on the six months I spent in the office and am extremely appreciative for the experience. It showed me exactly what I *didn't* want to do with my career. It has made me more grateful for all that I have now. There truly are no "bad" experiences in life, only ones that help us grow and learn. It just so happens that some experiences are more enjoyable than others.

The Move to Mayberry

After pouring Slurpees for a couple of months, I heard about a dental practice in Keystone Heights, a one-stoplight (literally) town about forty minutes from Gainesville, which needed a dentist. Being $125,000 in debt and a tad bored, I decided to make the move to Mayberry. (Remember Mayberry—the fictional hometown of *The Andy Griffith Show* on TV?)

The pace in the Keystone office was slower, to say the least. Instead of running between five treatment rooms, seeing sixty patients a day and never having time for lunch, I strolled between two treatment rooms, saw and chatted with six patients a day, and almost always had time for a leisurely lunch. But here's what blew my mind: At the end of the day, with an average fee schedule, my production was three times higher in the small-town office! Best of all, I enjoyed dentistry again.

At the same time, I began studying which physicians were doing well. I discovered it was the dermatologists and cosmetic surgeons. For the most part, they do elective procedures not covered by insurance. I wanted to find a similar specialty in dentistry and quickly discovered it was cosmetic dentistry.

I had heard from several sources that LVI was the best place to receive cosmetic dentistry training. So I got another loan (my banker was loving me by now!) and took my eight-months pregnant wife with me to Vegas. On the first day of the program, LVI's founder, Bill Dickerson, asked everyone to tell the group about their offices. When it was my turn to speak, I stood up and said, "I have no office, no employees, and a fistful of loans. I'm here to learn how to do fantastic cosmetic dentistry." He thought I was a little crazy, but sanity isn't all its cracked up to be.

Two Practices, Two More Loans, and One Cot in the Corner

I worked in the Keystone Heights practice for almost two years before obtaining a loan to purchase it. In the meantime, with another $150,000 loan from my bank, I bought an office in Gainesville that used to belong to an endodontist. Five days a week, I worked mornings in the Keystone office and afternoons in the Gainesville office.

I had only one lady helping me in Gainesville. Because money was really tight, I stayed in the office most evenings doing lab work, scrubbing instruments, keeping the books, and developing marketing plans. I would even sleep there on a small cot for weeks at a time. Luckily, Kim was a second-year dental student at the time, so she was busy studying.

I had a clear vision of the dental practice I wanted to create. I wanted a high-end, cosmetically-oriented, true fee-for-service practice. I can't ever remember a time when I thought I might fail. I always knew it would work. Having a crystal-clear and compelling dream is so important in life. My vision gave me the willpower I needed to keep going when things were a little tough.

Goodbye Mayberry, Hello Dream Office

Because the office in Gainesville was going so well, I was able to sell the practice in Keystone Heights. After three years in the Gainesville location, we outgrew the space and decided to build a new office.

I did what everyone told me not to do—opened a high-end cosmetic practice in a college town saturated with dentists. Kim and I decided to design a completely new facility that would look nothing like a dental office. We wanted the sights, sounds, smells, tastes, and touches in the new office to create a unique experience for everyone who walked through its doors. I believe we succeeded as the photos on the following page illustrate.

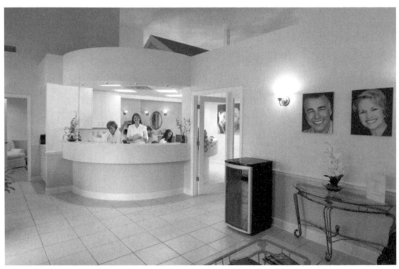

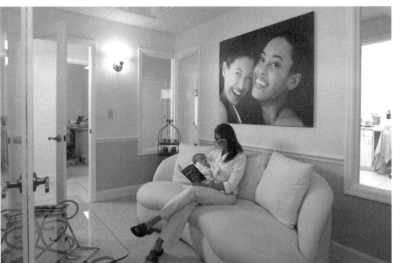

The interior of Art's office.

I must have done something right. I marketed the heck out of the practice, never signed up for an insurance plan or filed an insurance claim, put together a team of people who provided premium customer service, and received pre-payment in full for almost every case we started. In the second year, I netted far more than the average U.S. dentist. By the fifth year, we crossed the $2 million mark, and my net had increased 250% while I worked the equivalent of three days a week. We schedule people from 9 A.M. to 3 P.M. with no lunch break.

Three Important Choices

Later in the book, you will learn Empowering Belief #1: My Success Is a Choice. Our successes to date are primarily due to three important choices.

The first was our choice to attend LVI. We will always be grateful to Bill Dickerson for teaching us to stand up to the people and institutions that perpetuate the status quo. Bill also taught us it's desirable to make a great living being a dentist. We deserve to earn high incomes when we deliver high-quality dental care.

The second was our choice to form a business relationship. We can still remember sitting together at an LVI instructor's meeting in Vail, Colorado, and discussing how we would team up to help dentists become more successful.

The third was our choice to attend a James Arthur Ray program. He's one of the people featured in the book and DVD, *The Secret*. James helped us define our life purposes and taught us how to create Harmonic Wealth® in all aspects of our lives. There are vitally important lessons we all need to learn. We just have to be ready, find a teacher who resonates with us, learn the lessons, and take action based on our knowledge. James was and is that teacher for us.

Conclusion

We didn't describe our journeys and disclose our practice information to impress you. We did it to impress upon you that you can achieve anything in your life when you hold beliefs that empower you and then enthusiastically take action.

As you've learned, our journeys weren't always easy. There were numerous hills and valleys, twists and turns on the paths to where we now stand. Your journey will have similar challenges. And you will find, just as we did, that the rewards you receive will make the journey worthwhile.

Book Preview

This book is divided into three sections. In Section 1 you will explore The Power of Belief. You will discover how your empowering beliefs fly like a boomerang and return to create your professional and personal lives.

In Section 2, The Ten Empowering Beliefs, you will discover how ten beliefs silently guide the choices you make and the results you achieve—in your practice and your life.

In Section 3, Harmonic Wealth®, you will learn how to set SMART goals that lead to the future you desire and deserve and how to create that future. So let's get started. Turn the page now and begin to unearth a treasure of enormous value—The Power of Belief.

Section 1

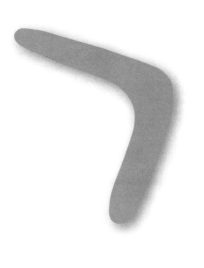

The Power of Belief

Two students are sitting on opposite sides of a small table. A teacher approaches and places a card between them. The card has one word printed on it. The teacher asks student A on the left side of the table, "What word is printed on the card in front of you?"

Student A answers, "The word is 'TRUE.'"

The teacher asks student B on the right side of the table, "What word is printed on the card in front of you?"

Student B answers, "The word is 'FALSE.'"

The students are thoroughly confused. They ask the teacher, "How can this be? We're both looking at the same word."

The teacher replies, "It is true. You are looking at the same card, but you are looking at it from two different perspectives. The same is true of life. How you look at the world determines what you see."

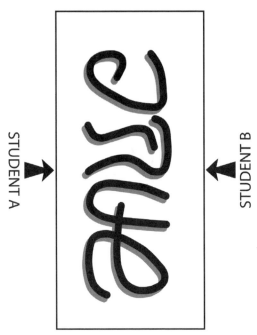

The poet John Milton agreed with the teacher's words when he wrote, "The mind is its own place and in itself can make a heaven of hell and a hell of heaven." William Shakespeare concurred when he penned, "There is nothing either good or bad but thinking makes it so."

Your mind is a thought factory. And the most powerful thoughts, the ones that determine how you look at the world, are your beliefs. In this section, we will explore the wonderful world of beliefs. In the first chapter you will take a ride around The Belief Cycle to see how it creates the actions you take and the results you get. In the second chapter you will learn how your thoughts attract that which is thought of. In the third chapter you will learn how to transform your limiting beliefs.

We believe in the power of the material you are about to discover. It has created the lives and practices you read about in the introduction. We know it will do the same for you. Take another step now by reading the next chapter, The Belief Cycle.

1

The Belief Cycle

Ready for a brief quiz? Fill in the blanks in the two sentences below. There are no right or wrong answers. Just write what you truly believe.

The world is a _____ **place.**

The world is full of _____ **people.**

Intrigued? We'll come back to your answers later in this chapter. Meanwhile, let's examine how your beliefs create your world. Beliefs are slippery little devils. Even though they are constantly careening around your cranium, they're difficult to grab hold of and examine. The working definition of belief we will use has three parts:

1. A belief is any thought held as true.

2. A belief is a connection between two entities.

3. A belief defines whether this connection is positive, neutral, or negative.

As an example, if you believe "My dental staff is a bunch of whiney slackers," you:

1. Hold that statement as true.

2. Connect your staff with the description "whiney slackers."

3. Define the connection as negative.

If you believe "My dental team is a group of wonderful, hard-working people," you:

1. Hold that statement as true.

2. Connect your team with the description "wonderful, hard-working people."

3. Define the connection as positive.

The Five Belief Cycle Elements

What's truly fascinating is that the two beliefs described above kick off a specific cycle of events that return like a boomerang to create the believer's world. The Belief Cycle has five elements: Belief, Focus, Emotion, Action, and Results.

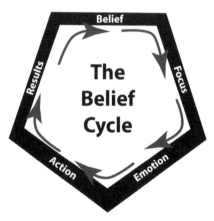

To examine The Belief Cycle in action, let's use the example of one of the world's greatest inventors, Thomas Edison. One of Edison's most famous inventions was the first commercially practical incandescent light bulb, which we still use today. One of his empowering beliefs, in paraphrased form, was, "There is no such thing as failure. We learn something from every experiment we do."

Let's go back in time to Edison's Menlo Park, New Jersey, laboratory in 1879 and watch that belief in action. One of Edison's people has just completed an experiment that didn't work out as intended.

1. *What did Edison believe?* "There is no such thing as failure. We learn something from every experiment we do."

2. *What did Edison focus on?* He focused on what they learned from the experiment. That learning would aid them in their next experiment.

3. *How did Edison respond to the event emotionally?* Was he discouraged? Was he upset? Heck, no! He was excited because he knew they were one step closer to their goal.

4. *What action did he take?* He directed his people to do another experiment using their new knowledge.

5. *What result did he get?* His team invented the first commercially practical incandescent light bulb. How many separate experiments did Edison's team conduct to achieve success? More than 10,000! Edison's belief and his ability to convey that belief to his team gave them all the encouragement they needed to keep going until they reached their goal.

"Genius is one percent inspiration and ninety-nine percent perspiration."

—Thomas Edison

But wait, there's more! How did their light bulb success affect Edison's original belief that "There is no such thing as failure. We learn something from every experiment we do"? It strengthened the belief and propelled him to obtain 1,093 U.S. patents on numerous other inventions such as the phonograph. That's the power of The Belief Cycle. It's self-perpetuating.

Rut and Roll

Have you ever been in a rut? If so, the rut could have begun with any element of The Belief Cycle. Let's say you're in an unresourceful emotional state that was sparked by an unexpected, negative event in your life. You stop taking important actions in your life. The results you achieve diminish proportionally. The lousy results cause you to believe that things aren't going to work out the next time. You focus on how your life is going to be adversely affected, which makes you feel worse— and the in-a-rut cycle keeps spinning along.

Our favorite definition of a rut is "a coffin with the ends kicked out." Many of the dentists we talk to in our seminars feel trapped in a rut. They want out, but they don't know how to do it. They always want us to tell them what to *do*. They never ask us what they need to *believe*. They always focus on the *outer*—their behavior. They never focus on the *inner*—their belief systems. That's why we wrote this book—to give you the *inner* resources you need to create *outer* results in your dental practice and life.

Conversely, have you ever been on a roll? You believe you can accomplish an outcome. You focus on all the resources you need to achieve the outcome. You feel energized. You take enthusiastic action. You achieve sensational results, which reinforce your belief, and the on-a-roll cycle keeps spinning along. We're on a roll in our practices and our lives right now. We're committed to showing you how to do the same.

Self-Fulfilling Prophecy

The Roman poet Virgil wrote, "They can because they think they can." How true. The corollary to this belief is "They can't because they think they can't." When people believe they can't accomplish a task, they focus on all the reasons they won't succeed. They feel discouraged. They take no or half-hearted action. They don't achieve their desired results, which reinforces their original belief.

We see this all the time in dentistry, in which there are unwritten rules that dentists are directly and indirectly taught. These unwritten rules place severe boundaries on dentists' beliefs of what's possible in their practices. As a result, they put themselves in tiny boxes, provide average care, and never feel fulfilled in their profession. What a tragedy that is!

"No matter what you believe, you're right."

Here's an example of what we're talking about: There is an unwritten rule in dentistry that says "You must play the insurance game according to the insurance companies' rules." If you believe you can't play the game with different rules, you focus on all the reasons it can't be done. You feel discouraged. You won't take action and keep getting the same old results, which reinforce your original belief. Spooky, isn't it?

In our *Achieving Extreme Success* seminars, we help dentists and their teams change the unwritten rules by which they play the dentistry game. *And* we teach them the action steps to become successfully insurance independent. People who just believe and are excited but don't know what they're doing are dangerous. We want you to believe *and* know what you're doing.

Here's an interesting question to ponder: What would happen if all of us changed our beliefs about playing the insurance game and stood up to the eight-hundred-pound insurance company gorilla in the room? Would the bullying gorilla leave our house?

Here's an example of *positive* self-fulfilling prophecy. An unwritten rule in dentistry is "the tighter your schedule is packed and the further you're completely booked into the future, the better you will do at the end of the year." We don't believe that at all, and our experiences confirm our belief. We believe a few comprehensive cosmetic and restorative cases lightly scheduled improve our net profit. We believe it's good to have holes in the schedule three weeks out. We can give that time to people who want their comprehensive dentistry done now. As a result of our belief, we focus on attracting people who already desire comprehensive cosmetic and restorative dentistry. We focus on making it easy for them to come to our offices and learn what's possible. We focus on getting the training that allows us to provide high-quality dentistry and five-star service. As a result, we feel fantastic as we provide the kind of care that produces outstanding results for patients and ourselves, thereby reinforcing our empowering beliefs. It all begins with belief. It all begins with you heeding a personal version of Virgil's sage advice: "You can because you think you can."

Back to the Beginning

In the beginning of this chapter, you filled in the blanks in two sentences. If you didn't do it then, please do it now.

The world is a _____ *place.*

The world is full of _____ *people.*

We had you complete this exercise to illustrate a key point about your belief system. That key point is this: Your beliefs about the world and the people in it return like a boomerang to create your personality. Let us explain. You can have beliefs in three general areas:

1. *Beliefs about Self*: These beliefs typically begin with the words "I am…." Beliefs about self constitute your identity. We will explore identity further in the chapters on Core

Belief #3: I'm the Best Dentist in the Area and Core Belief #7: I'm Here to Serve My Team and Patients.

2. *Beliefs about Other People*: These beliefs typically begin with the words "People are…."

3. *Beliefs about the World*: These beliefs typically begin with the words "The world is…."

For example, Mike believes "The world is a rotten place and is full of disgusting people." What do you think Mike focuses on all day long at work? The rotten world and all the disgusting people, of course. What TV programs does he watch when he comes home? Mike probably watches the local news so he can see all the rotten and disgusting things that happened during the day. Then he watches a thirty-minute celebrity gossip program so he can learn all the rotten and disgusting things the movie stars and athletes have done that week. Next, it's a series of shows like *Jerry Springer* and *Cops*. Mike finishes off his evening with more local news in case there's been another convenience store robbery since the 6 P.M. newscast.

Focusing on all this garbage makes Mike feel rotten and disgusted, which propels him to withdraw from most of the world and have a series of "Isn't it terrible" conversations with people who share his beliefs. These actions lead to lousy results at work and an unfulfilling personal life, which reinforce his belief that the world is a rotten place full of disgusting people. The Belief Cycle strikes again.

Here's the other side of the coin. In some of our seminars we have the entire audience complete the

The world is a _____ *place.*

The world is full of _____*people.*

exercise. Then we ask the group, "Who is one person on your dental team you love to work with? This person is always pleasant, helpful, and caring. This person just radiates love and happiness." There are always members of a dental team who enthusiastically raise their hands and shout out a person's name. Then we go to the person and ask her to read the two words she wrote in the blanks. One hundred percent of the time, what kinds of words do you think this person used? They're always words like "wonderful," "lovely," "nice," "great," "terrific," and "fantastic."

The moral of the story: *Your beliefs about the world and the people in it return to create the kind of person you are.*

Take a look at the two words you added to the blanks. If they aren't the most flattering words on the planet, don't feel bad. Your beliefs about the world and the people in it have been shaped by your life experiences. Luckily, it's never too late to transform these beliefs. We'll show you how to do that in a future chapter.

Einstein's Question

Albert Einstein believed the most important question a person could ask is, "Is the world a friendly place?" Now, do you see why this is such an important question? If your answer is "No," your belief will return like a boomerang to make you less friendly.

If your answer is "Yes," your belief will return like a boomerang to make you more friendly.

Conclusion

In this chapter, you discovered how your beliefs return to you with astounding accuracy through The Belief Cycle. This is only one half of The Power of Belief. The other half is the subject of the next chapter, The Law of Attraction. I have faith you will turn the page and keep reading now.

2

The Law of Attraction

This chapter builds on the last one. The previous chapter revealed how your thoughts lead to *action*. This chapter shows how your thoughts lead to *attraction*.

The Law of Attraction states that everything coming into your life is attracted by your thoughts. As an example, if you believe the world is an unfriendly place, you will consistently focus on all the unfriendly people, events, and things in your world. You will then automatically attract unfriendly people, events, and things into your life.

Conversely, if you believe the world is a friendly place, you will consistently focus on all the friendly people, events, and things in your world. You will then automatically attract friendly people, events, and things into your life.

It doesn't matter whether you believe in the Law of Attraction or know how it operates. The Law of Attraction is creating your entire life experience right now. It doesn't matter where you came from, who you are, or where you live. The Law of Attraction is at your service 24/7.

We're not certain whether anyone knows for sure how the Law of Attraction works. Big deal. We really don't know how gravity works, but we use it to play catch with our kids. One explanation of how the Law of Attraction operates is that every thought you generate vibrates at a unique frequency. As you hold the thought in your mind, the vibration is sent out into the universe and connects with all the resources that have the same frequency. When it comes to The Law of Attraction, like attracts like.

> "All that we are is the result of what we have thought."
>
> **—Buddha**

It's easy to extend the Buddha's comment to say, "All that we will be is the result of what we are now thinking." As we write this book, we're thinking about creating a document that will dramatically enhance your life. We have the Table of Contents taped to our monitors. We're writing 1,000–2,000 words a day. At times, we really don't know what we're going to write next. And some unique idea *always* pops into our minds. Thomas Edison once said, "Ideas come from space." We agree.

Your Wish Is My Command

The story of Aladdin, his magic lamp, and the Genie has been around for centuries and is told in one form or another in most cultures. It is the perfect metaphor for The Law of Attraction.

- Aladdin discovers the magic lamp and dusts it off.
- You discover The Law of Attraction and learn how it works.

- Aladdin rubs the magic lamp and out pops a Genie.
- You don't have to do anything. The Universal Power* is always there for you.

- Aladdin makes a wish and the Genie says, "Your wish is my command."
- You make a wish, and the Universal Power says, "Your wish is my command."

- Aladdin's wish comes true, and he has two more wishes in his future.
- Your wish comes true, and you have unlimited wishes in your future.

* People use different names for the Universal Power. God, Life, Mother Nature, Allah, Supreme Being, Brahma, and Jehovah are common examples. Please use the name that works for you as we're not here to place our label over your name.

The Universal Power

The Universal Power assumes you're wishing for everything you think about. The Universal Power doesn't judge your wish. It only answers it. After hearing your wish, the Universal Power immediately begins to manipulate the universe through people and events and provides you with the resources you need to make your wish come true. The more often you express your wish emotionally with thoughts and images, the more frequently and completely the Universal Power exerts its force.

There may be a gestation period before your wish hatches, however. Sometimes it takes a while for the resources you need to reach your doorstep. Sometimes it takes you a while to recognize the resources. Sometimes it takes a period of time for you to use the resources to craft your wish. Sometimes the Universal Power just wants to make sure you truly believe in your wish. But the Universal Power always answers, "Your wish is my command."

"God's delays are not God's denials."

—Dr. Robert Schueller

Think about What You Want

To make your wishes come true, it's vital that you focus mentally on what you want, not what you don't want. This sounds simple in theory, but sometimes it's more difficult to do in the real world. Here's a fictitious example of what we're talking about. Money is tight at the office for Dr. Bitchalot. His expenses are steadily increasing, but his gross income is holding steady. His spouse has several projects around the house that "need" to be funded. His kids are going to private school, and the tuition just went up 13 percent. One of the cars needs repairs. He's taken out a series of ever-increasing second mortgages to stay ahead of the game.

If Dr. Bitchalot constantly thinks about his debt, the Universal Power hears him and responds, "Your wish is my command." Then it will give him more debt. If he focuses on needing more money, the Universal Power will continue to give him "needing more money." If he thinks about what he doesn't have (the empty half of the glass of water), the Universal Power will give him more emptiness.

So what should Dr. Bitchalot think about? He should focus on his desires. We will explain how to do that a little later with our NEO Approach to making dreams come true.

Use Your Emotions As a Signal

Sometimes it's difficult to know which of your thoughts do the best job of rubbing your magic lamp and directing the Universal Power to grant your wishes. It's impossible to monitor all your thoughts as you have about sixty thousand of them each day. Luckily, you have a built-in signal that will immediately tell you whether you're on track or not. That signal is your emotions. Negative emotions send the signal that you're telling the Universal Power what you *don't* want. Positive emotions send the signal that you're telling the Universal Power what you *do* want.

> "Pleasure is nature's test, her sign of approval.
> When man is happy, he is in harmony with himself
> and his environment."
>
> **—Oscar Wilde**

Here's an example of what we mean. If Dr. Bitchalot feels discouraged, that negative emotion is signaling him to stop thinking about his problem and to start thinking about what he desires—the financial freedom that comes with netting $250,000 a year.

The NEO Approach to Making Your Desires Come True

We believe there is a three-step approach to making your desires come true. We call it the NEO Approach. The three steps are:

1. **N**ame Your Desire
2. **E**xpect Your Desire
3. **O**wn Your Desire

Name Your Desire

Give your desire a name. Make sure it's what you what, not what you don't want. Dr. Bitchalot's desire is the financial freedom that comes with netting $250,000 a year. Naming your desire is the spark that points you in the direction of the desire.

Here are other examples of naming your desire:

- "I desire a special person to share my life with."
- "I desire peace in our home."
- "I desire to write a book."
- "I desire the wisdom to help my child through a tough time in her life."
- "I desire a nursing degree."

You can't stop with just naming your desire because the Universal Power will give you more of what you're thinking about. In Dr. Bitchalot's case, the Universal Power will give him more of desiring financial freedom.

Expect Your Desire

Now that you've named your desire, expect it will come into your life. Expectation is a belief that connects you with your desire. You can't be half-hearted with your expectation. You can't expect your desire sometimes and not expect it other times. You can't expect it for a day or so and then give up. You must expect your desire totally, all the time.

You can't stop with just expecting your desire because the Universal Power will give you more of what you're thinking about. In Dr. Bitchalot's case, the Universal Power will give him more of expecting financial freedom.

Own Your Desire

Now that you've named your desire and expect that it will come into your life, you must own it. Owning your desire is the magnet that attracts the desire into your life. There are four mental methods you can use to own your desire:

1. Be grateful for what you have.

2. Create an ownership statement.

3. Vividly imagine having your desire.

4. Feel it.

1. Be Grateful for What You Have

Before you think about what you desire, it's vital to be grateful for what you already have and your ability to acquire more. Using the time-honored "half-full or half-empty" glass of water metaphor, when you express your gratitude for the half-full portion of your glass, the Universal Power will notice and be willing to fill up the rest of your glass. Conversely, when you focus on the portion of the glass that is half empty, the Universal Power will notice that too and give you more of what you're thinking about—emptiness.

Dr. Bitchalot shouldn't think about the gap between what he is currently making and what he wants to make. He should focus on the money he is making, his ability to earn more, and the tremendous opportunity dentists have to "set their own salaries."

> "Good thoughts bear good fruit, bad thoughts bear bad fruit—and man is his own gardener."
>
> **—James Allen**

2. Create an Ownership Statement

After expressing your gratitude for what you have, it's time to create a short ownership statement written in the *present* tense. Dr. Bitchalot's statement could read, "I am happily earning $250,000 a year and enjoying financial freedom." The two key words that begin the best ownership statements are "I am."

3. Vividly Experience Having Your Desire

Mental method #3 may be the most powerful one of the four. Albert Einstein phrased it best when he said, "Imagination is everything. It is the preview of life's coming attractions." We mentally process information with our five senses, not words. To write the story of your life from this moment on, you need to intensely experience having your desire by creating mental movies that harness the power of all five of your senses.

See—Instead of watching a movie of yourself acting out your desire, vividly experience the visual portion of your desire through your own eyes. See the world around you as big, bright and colorful, with tons of exciting action.

Hear—Acutely hear all the sounds and voices around you. Turn up the volume and excitement level of the sounds. Hear what people are telling you about your achievement.

Smell—Smell all the wonderful odors that are in the environment with your desire in place. Enjoy the sweet smell of success.

Taste—Taste the foods you will enjoy as you live your desire. Get a taste of all the pleasure you are experiencing.

Touch—Touch the people and things around you. Feel the hugs of the special people in your life.

4. Feel It

As you experience your desire and create a vivid mental movie, it's vital that you intensely feel it as if it were happening right now. As you take your morning shower, close your eyes, run the mental movie in your mind, and feel how fantastic it is to be living your dream. Do the same thing several times during the day. As you're lying in bed just before you fall asleep, vividly imagine yourself living your desire and feel the joy of its achievement.

Now, It's Time to Act

The Universal Power hears your wish and sends resources (in the form of people, ideas, and opportunities) into your life that you need to make your wish come true. Now, you must learn from the people, capture the ideas, and take advantage of the opportunities. In other words, *you must take action when the resources appear.* The Bible says, "Faith without works is dead." Most other holy books give similar advice. The following story illustrates what we mean.

A man is trapped in his home during a devastating flood. As the flood waters rise, the man climbs onto his roof and prays to God to rescue him. Just then, people in a boat come along and shout to him, "Jump in. We'll take you to safety."

The man replies, "No, I've prayed to God, and God's coming to rescue me."

A few minutes later, the flood waters creep even closer to the man. A rescue helicopter appears overhead and dangles a ladder for the man to climb up. The man shouts up, "Go away! I've prayed to God, and God's coming to rescue me."

A few minutes later, the flood waters are almost ready to wash the man off his roof. A second boat appears at the last second. A woman in the boat yells at the man, "You must get off your roof now! Hop aboard!"

For a third time, the man replies, "I have prayed to God, and God's coming to rescue me."

A few minutes later, the man is swept of his roof and drowns in the swirling flood water. He ascends to heaven, walks through the pearly gates, and confronts God. The man says, "God, what happened down there? I had faith in you. I prayed to you. And you never came to rescue me. I'm so disappointed."

God replied, "Hey, dude, I sent you two boats and a helicopter, but you chased them away and just sat there. You should've done something."

The moral of the story? The Universal Power will send you the resources you desire. To recognize these resources, you *must* pay attention. To the extent that you do not pay attention, you will pay with pain in your life. To the extent that you do pay attention, you will experience pleasure in your life.

After you pay attention to and recognize the resources, you need to use them actively. We call this "doing the work." And when you do the work, you will receive the benefits.

There's a Reason

There's a reason people show up and events occur in your life. The people and events appearing to be bad are there to teach you valuable lessons. One of the best things that ever happened to Art was working in the corporate dental office after dental school. It didn't seem too wonderful at the time, but the lessons he learned there shaped his view of the way he wanted to practice. Likewise, if you're unhappy with the way your dental practice is going, that's a signal to change your thinking and actions. We refer to these seemingly negative experiences as "growth opportunities."

The people and events appearing to be good are there to provide you with resources. We learned about the LVI resource at the same time in our careers. We attended the same first program—even though we didn't know it at the time. We sat down and talked at the LVI instructors' meeting in Vail. We quickly realized we were valuable resources for each other.

There's a reason we wrote this book. There's a reason you're reading it. You attracted the book and our ideas into your life. Our question to you is this: "Are you going to use the resources in the book—or not?" Don't be like the guy sitting on his roof in the flood. Pay attention. Answer the call. Do the work. You will be glad you did.

Conclusion

Our teacher, James Arthur Ray, is constantly reminding us to think, feel, and act. This is what James calls "going three for three."® In these first two chapters, you learned how your beliefs direct your thoughts, which create your feelings, which in turn lead to your actions. If your beliefs aren't producing the thoughts, feelings, and actions that lead to your wishes, you need to change them. Luckily, that's the subject of the next chapter, How to Transform Your Beliefs.

3

How to Transform Your Beliefs

In Chapter 1, you discovered the power of The Belief Cycle. You learned how beliefs direct your focus, which creates your emotions. Your emotions then spark specific actions, which produce your results in life. The results reinforce the original belief, and The Belief Cycle spins merrily along.

In Chapter 2, you learned how beliefs act as the commander of your brain. Behind the scene, they determine your thoughts. Then, according to the Law of Attraction, the Universal Power detects your thoughts, says "Your wish is my command," and gives you more of what you're thinking about.

With your beliefs exerting so much power over your life, it's vitally import to identify your limiting beliefs and transform them into empowering ones. After you've done that, you will want to identify additional empowering beliefs in your role models and install them in your mind. Let's start with your limiting beliefs.

Transforming Limiting Beliefs into Empowering Ones

Beliefs are remarkably resistant to change because people tend to focus on worldly evidence that reinforces their beliefs. To overcome this, you will need to develop and follow a specific, five-step plan for transforming a limiting belief into an empowering one:

1. Identify your limiting belief.
2. Produce motivation to drop your limiting belief.
3. Create a new, empowering belief.
4. Experience the future with your empowering belief in place.
5. Reinforce your empowering belief.

Step 1—Identify Your Limiting Belief

Not surprisingly, limiting beliefs are the ones that don't serve you. Sometimes your upbringing, past experiences, professional training, and the media you listen to, read, and watch teach you limiting beliefs. So don't feel bad if you have a few. We all do. The secret is to identify and change them. Because belief patterns are learned, they can be unlearned.

Some of your limiting beliefs are conscious ones, so you can identify them fairly easily. To get you started on your conscious limiting belief hunt, here are some we routinely see in dentists:

- "Dentists shouldn't make a lot of money."
- "If I work fewer hours, my income will go down."
- "I can't raise my fees. People will think I'm greedy."
- "The more people I see, the better I do."
- "A jam-packed schedule is good."
- "It's good for the schedule to be filled far into the future."
- "People don't do comprehensive dentistry in my area."
- "I can't ever find good people to work in my practice."
- "I can't change now. I'm too old/too set in my ways/too well established."

- "Only certain people can have high-quality, higher-fee practices."
- "I'm the boss. My staff works for me."
- "I have to be everybody's dentist."
- "I have to go along with the other dentists in my area."
- "I have to play it safe."
- "That won't work in my area."
- Any belief beginning with, "I can't…."
- Any belief beginning with, "There's no way…."

Some of your limiting beliefs are buried and are harder to identify. It takes some digging to unearth them. Here are two ways you can do it:

1. Whenever you feel a negative emotion that doesn't serve you, ask yourself this question: "What would I have to believe to feel this way?" As an example, if you feel fear when you consider raising your fees 10%, you may hold a belief that "People in my area won't pay that much." Incidentally, fear isn't always bad. I hope you're fearful of jumping off a ten-story building. That fear supports you.

2. Whenever you take an action that doesn't serve you or don't take an action that would serve you, ask yourself this question: "What would I have to believe to act this way?" For example, if you're spending fifty hours a week at the office, you may hold the belief, "To make more money, I have to work more" or "I have to be everybody's dentist."

Using the information above as a guide, identify one of your limiting beliefs and write it on the lines below.

_____

_____

Step 2—Produce Motivation to Drop Your Limiting Belief

When it comes to changing them, beliefs can be incredibly stubborn. After all, they've been controlling your behavior for better or worse for years. Some people change their beliefs only after having a life-threatening experience such as a heart attack. We don't recommend waiting for something like that to happen.

We do recommend that you imaginarily produce an experience similar to the one Ebenezer Scrooge had on Christmas Eve when he was visited by three ghosts. We will walk you through the Scrooge experience using a common limiting belief, "A jam-packed schedule is good." Then, you will go through the same experience using the limiting belief you just wrote.

First, close your eyes and vividly imagine yourself being visited by the Ghost of Jam-Packed Schedule Past. This ghost transports you back in time to several situations where the limiting belief led to actions that were detrimental to you. Imagine several painful past experiences where your jam-packed schedule affected the quality of care you delivered; or where your jam-packed schedule drove you nuts; or where your jam-packed schedule led you to miss an important personal or family event. Feel in your gut the pain the jam-packed schedule has created in the past.

Now, vividly imagine yourself being visited by the Ghost of Jam-Packed Schedule Present. Experience what it is like now to go through day after day of running from room to room. Turn the volume up on all the sights, sounds, tastes, smells, and touches. Feel the pain your limiting belief is causing right now.

The Ghost of Christmas Future was the one who really scared the Dickens out of Scrooge. The Ghost was a grim specter who didn't speak. He was clothed in a long black robe. The only visible part of his body was a single hand, which pointed to scenes of all the dreadful events that would surely happen if Scrooge didn't change. The scene that had the most impact was the one of the Cratchit family minus Tiny Tim.

You need to do the same. With your eyes still closed, vividly imagine yourself being visited by the Ghost of Jam-Packed Schedule Future. Be with the Ghost as he points to scenes that will surely happen if you don't change your "a jam-packed schedule is good" belief now. See scenes of how the limiting belief will affect the quality of care you give, your health, your family relationships, and your joy for life. See and feel how your limiting belief will adversely impact loved ones. Don't hold back. Feel the pain. You can experience a little pain now or massive pain later if you don't change.

Now, imaginarily create a past, present and future Scrooge experience using the limiting belief you wrote previously. This will give you the motivation you need to change it.

Step 3—Create a New, Empowering Belief

Now that you're motivated to drop your limiting belief, you must replace it with a new, empowering one. Otherwise, a vacuum is created; and who knows what random belief might be sucked into the empty space. For the example we've been using, you could transform the "a jam-packed schedule is good" belief to "a light schedule filled with longer, comprehensive procedures is best for everyone."

On the lines below, write the newly created empowering belief to replace the old limiting belief you previously identified.

_____

_____

"The belief that becomes truth for me is the one that allows me the best use of my strength, the best means of putting my virtues into action."

—André Gide

Step 4—Experience the Future with Your Empowering Belief in Place

The Scrooge Experience provided the *pain* needed to change an old, limiting belief. Now, imaginarily give yourself the *pleasure* of a life with the new, empowering belief in place. Close your eyes and see all the pleasant scenes you will experience with your "a light schedule filled with longer, comprehensive procedures is best for everyone" empowering belief in place. See big, bright, and colorful positive images. Hear the happy voices of the people around you. Feel how wonderful it is to practice dentistry and live life with the new belief. Pay special attention to how your new belief will affect the people you care about.

Spend a few minutes doing this exercise. You will know you're doing it correctly when there's a smile on your face and you feel intense pleasure throughout your body.

"The secret of success is learning how to use pain and pleasure instead of having pain and pleasure use you. If you do that, you're in control of your life. If you don't, life controls you."

—Anthony Robbins

Step 5—Reinforce Your Empowering Belief

A new, empowering belief is like a thin strand of steel. It can be easily broken. The belief needs to be consistently reinforced. Each time it's reinforced, a new strand of steel is added to the original one. Through time, a thick and unbreakable steel cable is created. Here are four ways to reinforce your new, empowering belief:

• Create a Reinforcing Environment

It is absolutely vital that you create an environment that reinforces your new, empowering belief. If you don't, the thin strand of steel may be broken with the first bit of pressure. We see this happening all the time in dentistry. A dentist changes a belief and makes an improvement in her practice. Her team doesn't agree with the improvement and actively and/or passively resists it. The improvement doesn't stick. The behavior reverts back to "normal." The empowering belief is squashed. Worst of all, the dentist may never try something like that again because there's too much pain involved. Sound familiar?

Groups of local dentists can also be the belief squashers. Matt calls these groups "The Good Ol' Boys." The Good Ol' Boys don't like other dentists breaking the club rules and will actively and passively ostracize those who try. The Good Ol' Boys like conformity. It's more comfortable for them that way because they can continue playing their B game instead of learning the skills needed to play an A game.

We place enormous emphasis on creating a reinforcing environment in our practices. We know where we want our dental practices' buses to go. We only hire people who want to be on the bus and buy into our philosophy. If we discover people don't want to be on our bus, we give them a career adjustment so they can go ride on someone else's bus.

- Seek Out the Best Training

It's crucial that every member of your team (when we use the word "team," that includes you) receives the clinical and practice management training that will give you the skills you need to support your empowering belief. If your new, empowering belief is "a light schedule filled with longer, comprehensive procedures is best," then you will need the best training in comprehensive clinical dentistry. You will require marketing training so you can attract the kind of people who desire comprehensive dentistry. You need five-star service training so you can treat these people like they're guests in a Four Seasons Hotel. We believe the best training available is at the Las Vegas Institute. That's why our teams go there several times a year.

Another mistake we see dentists make is continually moving from one practice philosophy to another. You need to "dance with the one that brung ya" by selecting an office philosophy and sticking with it.

- Achieve Success Quickly

There are two things that will kill a new, empowering belief almost every time—procrastination and early failure. When you decide to take action on your new belief, do it quickly because the Universal Power loves speed. Most dentists spend their entire professional careers saying, "Someday I'll…." "Someday I'll stop double and triple booking myself" or "Someday I'll get advanced clinical training in cosmetic dentistry." Someday never comes. Don't procrastinate. Start now! Be one of the few who do, instead of the many who talk.

When you transform a belief and make a major improvement in your practice, set it up so you will be successful from the very beginning. Our good friend, Nate Booth, has written an insightful book called *Tiger Traits: 9 Success Secrets You Can Discover from Tiger Woods to Be a Business Champion.* In the book, Nate tells a story about one of Tiger's childhood golf instructors, Rudy Duran. Rudy established a "Tiger Par" for each hole the child played. If Tiger reached the green on an adult par four hole with six excellent shots, Rudy made Tiger Par for that hole an eight—six to reach the green plus two putts. So, from very early in Tiger's life, he was shooting par or better, which reinforced his belief that he was a fantastic golfer. As Tiger matured and could hit the ball farther, Rudy moved Tiger Par to seven, then six, then five, and finally four. As a result, Tiger was successful from the very beginning because he was always shooting par.

You need to do the same in your office. If you're moving from a jam-packed schedule full of lots of people to a light schedule filled with longer, comprehensive procedures, change your schedule for only half a day a week at first, then a full day, then a day and a half, etc.

• Teach What You've Learned to Others

The surest way to cement your new, empowering beliefs and the behaviors they produce is to teach what you've learned to others. Several times a year, both our teams teach our *Achieving Extreme Success* seminars in Las Vegas and other locations. After you've moved from having a jam-packed schedule full of lots of people to a light schedule filled with longer, comprehensive procedures, you can teach others to do the same.

With the empowering belief you wrote on the lines on a previous page, create a plan to reinforce the belief using the four ways outlined above.

Transform Another Limiting Belief

Now, transform another limiting belief into an empowering one using the same five-step technique:

1. Identify your limiting belief.
2. Produce motivation to drop your limiting belief.
3. Create a new, empowering belief.
4. Experience the future with your empowering belief in place.
5. Reinforce your empowering belief.

Identify Empowering Beliefs in Role Models

Now that you've transformed your limiting beliefs into empowering ones, it's time to identify empowering beliefs in the people you admire. We hope you have role models in dentistry and life—people whom you admire and want to emulate. When you find your role models, listen very carefully to what they say and watch closely what they do. Very often, their empowering beliefs will become evident. Pick their brains. Ask questions to discover what they're doing *and* how they're thinking.

In the Introduction, you read the story of Matt meeting Dr. David Philip at LVI. Matt learned from David this empowering belief: "Spending lots of quality time with your family and doing the kinds of dentistry you love are the two keys to a prosperous personal and professional life." Matt adopted David's empowering belief and uses it as a cornerstone for his life to this day.

One of Art's role models is Bill Dickerson. From him, Art learned and adopted the following empowering belief: "To create the practice of your dreams and to feel fulfilled in dentistry you must stand up to the people perpetuating the status quo."

So, who are your role models in and out of dentistry? List their names on a sheet of paper and after each name write the empowering beliefs and important life lessons you've learned from them. Your role models can be people you know, people you've met, people who have taught programs you've attended, and/or people who've written books you've read. It's also an excellent idea to write a letter to your role models expressing your gratitude for their ideas.

After you identify the empowering beliefs you want to adopt, complete Steps 4 and 5 described on previous pages—experience the future with your empowering belief in place and reinforce your empowering belief.

Conclusion

It never fails to happen. We talk to a group of dentists about making dramatic improvements in their practices and somebody always says, "Come on now. Let's be realistic about things. Not everybody can blah blah blah blah blah blah blah." When used that way, the word "realistic" really bothers us.

It's just a cop out that makes people feel okay about not going outside their comfort zone and doing something new. Realistic people adapt themselves to their view of the "real" world. As a result, they never move beyond what everybody else is doing in the "real" world and remain mired in the mud of mediocrity. "Realistic" is just another word for complacency. And complacency breeds mediocrity.

We're unrealistic and proud of it. We don't adapt to the world. We adapt the world to us. We know that all progress is due to unrealistic people. We want you to be unrealistic, too. That way we can change the face of dentistry together.

Enough of the preliminaries. It's time to present the empowering beliefs that have led to our practices' success. We know they can do the same for you. Turn the page to begin Section 2: The Ten Empowering Beliefs.

The Ten
Empowering Beliefs

As our *Achieving Extreme Success* seminar evolved, we identified the ten most important empowering beliefs that returned like a boomerang to create our successes in dentistry and life. Of course, there are hundreds of other empowering beliefs available for your use. The ten we present in this chapter are the ones that have worked best for us.

You may already hold some of the empowering beliefs. Some of them may sound foreign to you at first. Some of them you may never have considered. And all of them are worthy of your consideration.

In this section, we will devote one chapter to each of the ten beliefs. We will discuss the belief and illustrate its power in the dental office and in life. Then, if you choose to adopt the belief, we will give you several sample actions that exemplify and reinforce the belief. Here are the Ten Empowering Beliefs:

Belief #1:
My success is a choice.

Belief #2:
I receive from life what I give to life.

Belief #3:
I'm the best dentist in the area.

Belief #4:
To have different, I must do different.

Belief #5:
**People need to know what we do and
how we do it.**

Belief #6:
Staff is an infection; team is the cure.

Belief #7:
I'm here to serve my team and patients.

Belief #8:
I must make emotional connections with people.

Belief #9:
I think big in everything I do.

Belief #10:
It's an honor to be a dentist.

The first empowering belief is "My success is a choice." Make the correct choice right now. Look to the next page and continue reading.

4

Empowering Belief #1:
My Success Is a Choice

In the two chapters about The Belief Cycle and The Law of Attraction, you learned that the beliefs you *choose* to hold and the thoughts you *choose* to produce determine the emotions you feel, the actions you *choose* to take, and the resources you attract. These choices determine the path you take in life. When you come to one of the numerous forks in the path, your choices determine which direction you head. See, it's in your moments of choice that your future is determined.

One of our favorite quotes is by the American poet, Robert Frost. He wrote, "Two roads diverged in a wood, and I—I took the one less traveled by, And that has made all the difference." When two roads diverge in their woods, most dentists choose the road *most* traveled. As a result, they do what everybody else does, become instantly average, and receive average emotional and financial rewards from their profession.

How boring is that? We're asking you to join us on the road less traveled. To do that, you may need to say goodbye to a few friends. You will need to step outside your comfort zone and take a few calculated risks. You will need to stand up and dust yourself off if you trip over a rock in the road. But when you reach the mountaintop and look down on the valley where you used to be, you will feel a sense of accomplishment that will make the whole journey worthwhile. Your sense of accomplishment will be magnified tenfold when you share the joy with your fellow travelers. As an added bonus, if enough of us choose the road less traveled, it will become the road *most* traveled. Then, our entire profession will benefit.

You're off to a good start on your journey. You've chosen to buy this book. You've chosen to read this far. Good for you. You've already separated yourself from 95% of the dentists. There are many more choices ahead. Some will be easy. Some won't. We're glad you've chosen us to be your guides.

Two Types of Choices

There's no doubt we all start from different places in life. We have different natural talents, and we were raised in different environments. In addition, we desire to go different places in life. It stands to reason that if we start from different places and want to go in different directions, we're all on different paths.

We define success as the progressive movement down a unique path toward a personalized set of desires. It's important to realize that you don't have to *achieve* your desires to feel successful—only be moving toward them. The direction and speed you move (if you're moving at all) is determined by the thought and behavior choices you make.

Some of your choices move you closer to your desires. We call these Type A choices. Some of your choices move you away from your desires. We call these Type B choices. It was tempting to call the first set of choices the "right" choices and the second set the "wrong" choices, but that wouldn't be accurate.

Was it "wrong" for Art to choose to work for the corporate dental office after he graduated? After all, Art spent six months of his life practicing dentistry in almost the exact opposite way he is now. We believe it was one of the best choices Art ever made because it taught him early the valuable lesson, "This is *not* how I want to practice dentistry."

Type B choices are an important part of the twisty path to your desires as long as you learn a lesson from the choice and quickly make a new Type A choice. The following three people agree:

> "I am not discouraged because every wrong attempt discarded is another step forward."
>
> **—Thomas Edison**

> "There are no failures in life. There are only results."
>
> **—Anthony Robbins**

> "Things turn out best for people who make the best of the way things turn out."
>
> **—John Wooden**

Fear—The Choice Stomper

We believe that fear and the inaction it creates are the choice stompers. You can be the most talented and well-meaning dentist in the world, but if you're afraid to make the choices that move you down the path to your desires, you just sit on the bench of life and watch everybody else pass by. After a while, you close your eyes or look away because that makes you feel more comfortable. Some bench-sitters even try to discourage the people walking by. They want others on their bench, as misery loves company.

There was a study done by the ADA a few years ago that found almost 70 percent of practicing dentists would *not* choose dentistry as a profession if they had to do it all over again. Isn't that an amazing statistic? And very, very sad. Why would people spend huge chunks of their lives doing something they don't enjoy? Why don't they choose to make things better or get out of the profession? The answer to both those questions is fear. They fear making a "wrong" choice that will make life worse, or they fear the people around them will react negatively. As a result, they sit on the bench of life with a whole bunch of other fearful dentists and complain about how bad their practices and lives are.

So what's the antidote for this fear? It's the knowledge that fear is the signal for a growth opportunity. Then it's making a series of Type A and B choices that will enable you to zigzag your way to success.

> "My motto was always to keep swinging.
> Whether I was in a slump or feeling badly or
> having trouble off the field, the only thing to do
> was keep swinging."
>
> —Hank Aaron

Your Beliefs Determine a Set of Possible Actions

Just as there are two types of choices, there are two places on The Belief Cycle where you can choose—your beliefs and your actions. Your beliefs lead the way. Through The Belief Cycle, they determine a set of possible actions you could take. Here's an example of what we mean: In The Belief Cycle chapter we gave you two examples of beliefs that dentists might hold when it comes to the people they work with. The first was, "My staff is a bunch of whiney slackers." If dentists believe that, they will tend to *focus* on all the actions of their staff members that support this belief. That, in turn, will make them feel the *emotion* of disgust, which will lead to a set of possible *actions*. The doctors could choose to:

1. Do nothing about the situation other than complain to their dental friends. This seems to be the preferred choice in the dental profession.

2. Gripe to the staffs about their behavior and threaten drastic consequences if the behavior isn't improved. This is the ever-popular "The firings will continue until morale improves" approach. This choice would probably perpetuate more of the whiney, slacker behavior.

3. Create a positive plan of action to improve the situation, communicate the plan to the team, and follow through with the plan's implementation. This may improve the situation.

4. Give some or all of the staff a "career adjustment" and find new people who have better attitudes. This may improve the situation.

Action choices 1 and 2 are poor choices because they are almost guaranteed to make the situation worse. Action choices 3 and 4 are better choices because they may create a more harmonious and better functioning team.

We hope you see that we're not just talking about positive thinking. "My staff is a bunch of whiny slackers" isn't a positive belief. But it is a belief that could lead to improvement of the situation *if* the right action choices are made.

An Easy Choice?

It's easy to *say*, "My success is a choice." But if you continually give excuses for your lack of success, that means you don't really believe it. Check it out now by answering this question: "If you aren't as successful as you would like to be, what are the reasons this is so?" If your answers lie outside yourself (the insurance companies, the people in my community, my office staff, or my debt), that means you believe your lack of success is due to external factors. That may make you feel better in the moment ("Hey, it's not my fault!"), but it severely limits your choices in the future.

If your answers lie within yourself, you have empowered yourself to make your practice and life what you choose.

Stop reading this chapter now unless you firmly hold Empowering Belief #1:

My success is a choice.

If you don't have Empowering Belief #1 firmly planted in your mind, the following information will be absolutely useless to you because the actions presented won't match your beliefs.

If you don't hold Empowering Belief #1 and choose to change it now, return to the chapter on How to Transform Your Beliefs and follow the instructions. If you do believe "my success is a choice," read on.

Actions That Exemplify Empowering Belief #1

Below is a list of choices we believe are important to make. We have grouped them in two categories—professional and personal. If needed, we encourage you to add your own choices to both categories. We're just asking you to make your choices now. We're not asking you to develop a detailed plan to achieve them. In addition, don't over-analyze your choices by thinking about all the reasons the choice won't be successful. Just calmly and coolly choose the ways you want to run your practice and live your life. If you find this exercise difficult to do or if the word "choose" seems strange, congratulations—you really need to do the exercise.

Practice Choices

1. How many days do you choose to work per year? (Matt chooses to work 120 days. Art chooses to work one day less than Matt.)

2. How many hours do you choose to work per day?

3. What types of dentistry do you choose not to do anymore?

4. What types of dentistry do you choose to do more of?

5. How many hours of continuing education do you choose to take each year?

6. How many people do you choose to have working with you?

7. What kind of people do you choose to have walking in your door for care?

8. How do you choose to deal with the insurance companies?

9. How do you choose for your office to look?

10. On a scale of 1 to 10, how much do you choose to enjoy your time in the office?

11. How much do you choose to net in the next twelve months?

Life Choices

1. On average, how much time do you choose to spend each week with your partner?

2. How much time do you choose to spend each week with your family?

3. How much time do you choose to spend each week playing sports or exercising?

4. How much time do you choose to spend each week on hobbies and/or reading?

5. What type of home do you choose to live in?

6. What kind of toys do you choose to own?

7. How many weeks vacation do you choose to take each year?

8. How much money do you choose to save each year?

9. How much do you choose to donate to charities each year?

10. On a scale of 1 to 10, how much do you choose to enjoy life this year?

Conclusion

Answer this riddle: Seven frogs are sitting on a lily pad. Four choose to jump off. How many frogs remain on the lily pad?

If you said seven, you're right. Choosing to jump off and actually doing it are two completely different things. We hope you've chosen to jump off your lily pad onto a better one. That's what this section of the book is designed to do. The next section, Harmonic Wealth®, will help you safely and successfully make the leap.

In the meantime, keep building up your leg muscles by reading the next chapter about Empowering Belief #2: I receive from life what I give to life.

5

Empowering Belief #2:
I Receive from Life What I Give to Life

Giver Story #1—Jim Carrey

Actor and comedian Jim Carrey became interested in comedy as a little boy growing up in Ontario, Canada. At first he just tried to cheer up his mother, who was frequently in poor health and suffered from depression. Then it became something much more. In Jim's words, here's what happened: "I remember having this actual thought when I was seven or eight years old. *'I'm going to prove to my mother that I'm a miracle, and that her life is worth something.'*"

Wow! Did Jim's thought italicized above hit you the way it did us? Do you believe it's possible that one thought totally changed the direction of Jim Carrey's life? We believe it's not only possible but probable.

"I'm going to prove to my mother that I'm a miracle, and that her life is worth something" is an empowering belief if there ever was one. It led Jim to focus on his mother. It gave him emotional strength during some very difficult times. It signaled the Universal Power to give Jim the resources he needed to create hilarious comedy routines for her. The results were smiles and laughter from the woman he loved, which reinforced his belief that he was a miracle and her life was worth something.

Jim Carrey gave his mom the gift of laughter. Jim also received a very interesting by-product—the comedic perspective and comedy training that he would use to create his success in later years. Jim received from life what he gave to life. It's the same with all of us.

Jim's mom died in 1991 but lived to see him become a favorite in Toronto-area comedy clubs. After he moved to Los Angeles, she saw him on TV as one of the favorites on *In Living Color*. We have a feeling she died knowing Jim was a miracle and that her life was worth something.

> "There is no exercise better for the heart
> than reaching down and lifting people up."
>
> **—John Holmes**

Giver Story #2—Tiger Woods

Tiger Woods is well on his way to becoming the greatest golfer of all time. His parents, Earl and Tida, repeatedly said they raised Tiger to be a better person than he was a golfer. The two words that were frequently used in the Woods household were "share and care." The following story told by Earl illustrates the Woods family's "share and care" attitude.

If Tiger had wanted to be a plumber, I wouldn't have minded, as long as he was a hell of a plumber. Our goal was for him to be a good person. He's a great person. He always had a gentle heart. As a child, there was a time when Tiger collected coins, gold coins. They were his pride and joy. One day, after seeing a TV documentary, he came to me with the coins and said, "Dad, could you send these to the kids in Africa?" Now I think everything he has given, and will give, is kind of like those coins.

Today, Tiger earns about $100,000,000 a year on and off the course. That's a whole lot of gold coins. What isn't so well known is the extent to which he continues to give back. Tiger is grateful for the lessons he learned from his parents. He's grateful for the experiences he had playing junior golf. He's grateful for the education he received in school. At the age of thirty-two (most people wait until they're sixty-two), Tiger is giving back in the same areas for which he is grateful. In 2006 he opened his first 35,000-square-foot Tiger Woods Learning Center for kids, not far from his boyhood home in Anaheim, California. Washington, D.C., is the next city scheduled to receive a learning center.

So what is Tiger receiving from his gifts? He's definitely receiving the knowledge that he's making a major difference in thousands of kids' lives. He is also receiving the admiration and respect from millions of people of all ages and races around the world. It's no wonder that an unusually high percentage of people want Tiger to win the golf tournaments he enters.

Does the majority of people in your area admire and respect you as a dentist and as a person? Do they want your dental practice to do well? If not, you need to look very closely at your patterns of giving.

Who You're Attracting Is a Reflection of What You're Giving

As we travel around the country speaking to dental groups about building outstanding office teams, we occasionally have a dentist come up to us and say, "I can't find any good people in my area to work for me. It's been that way for years."

We don't say the following, but we're sure as heck thinking it: "Hey, maybe your practice sucks!" We know there are times when it's difficult to locate great team members. But if it's always like that, it's not them—it's you. Sorry to break the news, but great dental practices tend to attract great patients and great team members. Average dental practices tend to attract average people. Lousy dental practices tend to attract lousy people. Take a really close look at the patients and team members you're attracting, because they're a direct reflection of your practice and you.

Examples of Our Giving

The two of us are receiving tremendous amounts of emotional and financial rewards from our practices because we provide outstanding service and high-quality dentistry. We also give back to our communities in unique ways. The following are examples.

Pay It Forward

Matt and his wife, Ann, saw a program on Oprah called *Pay It Forward*. They made the choice to do the same thing in their community. In early December, they gave each team member $1,000 with the instruction to do something positive with the money for a total stranger. Each of the ten team members had five weeks to work their magic. What was really interesting was how the $10,000 turned into $50,000 as the team members recruited other people and companies to join them. One team member enlisted the electric company to add to her $1,000 to help people in need pay for their home power bills during the winter months.

Matt and Ann didn't publicize *Pay It Forward*. But guess what? The local media found out about it, and they received lots of positive PR.

Charity Cases

Both of us do two or more charity cases each year. Here's a key distinction: We pick our charities. They don't pick us. We choose the people who truly need some help but don't ask for it. As an example, Art has a wonderful woman in his practice who adopts fourteen to sixteen-year-old kids and raises them until they graduate from high school. She brought one of them who needed a ton of restorative and cosmetic dentistry into his office. After hearing what it would cost to do the case, she told Art, "I don't have much money right now, but I'll send you $50 a month if you can help this boy." Art's team decided this was just the kind of person who deserved charity.

Become the Change You Seek in Your World

Mahatma Gandhi said, "We must be the change we wish to see." Take Gandhi's advice. Don't wait for others to change first. Life doesn't work that way. If you want to receive more love in your life, give more love away first. If you want more happiness in your life, give more happiness away first. If you want more success in your dental practice, provide more high-quality dentistry first. If you want people to refer their family and friends, treat them with more kindness first. If you want to make more money, change your ideas about how a dental practice should operate first.

> "Money never starts the idea; it is the idea that starts the money."
>
> **—William Cameron**

Stop reading this chapter now unless you firmly hold Empowering Belief #2:

I receive from life what I give to life.

If you don't have Empowering Belief #2 firmly planted in your mind, the following information will be absolutely useless to you because the actions presented won't match your beliefs.

If you don't hold Empowering Belief #2 and choose to change it now, return to the chapter on How to Transform Your Beliefs and follow the instructions.

If you do believe "I receive from life what I give to life," read on.

Actions That Exemplify Empowering Belief #2

Below is a list of actions that exemplify Empowering Belief #2: I receive from life what I give to life. Jump off your lily pad by doing one or more of them right now. Your actions will allow you to give more to your patients, team, family, and community.

1. In the last chapter, you chose the types of clinical dentistry you enjoy doing for people. Research the resources that provide the best training and sign up for a course.

2. To say most dentists are poor business people would be the understatement of the century. The more successful your practice is, the more you can give to your community. Research the resources that provide the best practice management training and sign up for some coaching.

3. Don't forget making yourself a better person. Research the best relationship and personal development training and enroll in a course.

4. Be a mentor to someone in your area who is eager to learn what you know.

5. *Pay It Forward* with your team in your community.

6. Provide charity care for at least two individuals or families in your community. Make sure they don't pick you, but you pick them.

7. Be like Jim Carrey. Visit or volunteer at a location where people need to know that their lives are worth living. This could be a retirement or veterans home, a hospital, or a Boys and Girls Club.

8. Be like Tiger Woods. Identify the things for which you're grateful and give back in the same areas.

Conclusion

As you've noticed, the arrangement of this book is a little strange. In each chapter, we instruct you *not* to read the last part of the chapter if you don't hold the belief that is discussed in the first part of the chapter. We're not attempting to be confrontational when we do this. We're being practical. We're saving you some time.

Have you ever wondered why dentists and dental teams attend training programs, go back to their offices, and do nothing? A primary reason this occurs is the actions taught in the programs don't match the belief systems of the folks attending it. So when the people get back to the real world, they:

1. don't do anything, or

2. make a change but allow it to fizzle out after a day, a week, or a month because there isn't any belief foundation to support the change in behavior.

The above is another way of saying, "The change we intended to make wasn't important enough to spend the effort to make it happen. So things just fizzled out." We don't want you to fizzle. We want you to dazzle. And you can do that by adopting the ten empowering beliefs one at a time. The one you should check out now is Empowering Belief #3: I'm the best dentist in the area.

6

Empowering Belief #3:
I'm the Best Dentist in the Area

There's a lot more to Empowering Belief #3 than you may realize right now. On the surface, "I'm the best dentist in the area" appears to be just a statement or even a boast. In reality, it's a very special and particularly potent belief—one that emphatically describes your identity and states your personal brand. Sounds pretty philosophical, doesn't it? What we're talking about is ultra-practical. We'll discuss identity first and personal brand second.

Identity

The movie *Spiderman* ends with Peter Parker declaring his identity. "Whatever life holds for me, I will never forget these words: 'With great power, comes great responsibility.' This is my gift, my curse. Who am I? I'm Spiderman." At that moment, Peter has made a conscious decision to assume the identity of Spiderman.

As Peter Parker, he could live a normal life. He could make ends meet selling his photos to the *Daily Bugle* and be with his true love, the beautiful Mary Jane Watson. But Peter realized he possessed the ability to do so much more with his life, even if it meant sacrificing the safety of mediocrity and having a romantic relationship with Mary Jane. By choosing to be Spiderman, he could use his superpowers to make a difference, sometimes between life and death, for people every day. Peter knew who he was and what he had to do.

Like Spiderman, all dentists have identities whether they can consciously describe them or not. We believe we're the best restorative and cosmetic dentists in our areas. We also believe we change people's lives by changing their smiles. There isn't a doubt in our minds. There are lots of dentists who are better with kids. There are dentists who treat advanced periodontal disease better than we do. But when it comes to restorative and cosmetic dentistry, we're the best.

From the above discussion we hope you see that "I'm the best dentist in the area" applies to the type of dentistry you do. It doesn't just apply to restorative and cosmetic dentistry.

Personal Brand

Peter worried for Mary Jane's safety. He knew Spiderman's enemies would come after her in order to reach him. Thus, he made it very clear to Mary Jane that he could just be her friend. He spoke compassionately but firmly. Mary Jane didn't attempt to convince him otherwise. Peter's identity as Spiderman communicated much louder than his words ever could. As strange as it might sound to you now, Spiderman was a personal brand. So are we, and so are you.

Personal Brands Are Words and Emotions in Other People's Heads

We will talk about two different but closely related types of brands. Your personal brand is an extension of who you are (your identity). Your office brand is what your practice stands for. Both brands are visibly expressed to others by *what* you do and *how* you do it. With enough repetition, your personal and office brands become words and emotions in other people's minds.

Here are some examples: What words pop into your mind when you think of Southwest Airlines? Most people think of "cheap" and "fun." What one word pops into your mind when you think of FedEx? Was it "reliable"? What words pop into your mind when you think of Tiger Woods? How about the words "winner," "success," and "confidence?" In our geographic areas, the words that pop into people's minds when they think of us are "the best," "life-changers," and "expensive."

See, brands are nothing more than words and emotions stored in someone else's head. The good news is once the words and emotions are there, they have tremendous staying power. Contrary to popular opinion, brands are not names, logos, slogans, advertisements, and tag-lines—although these may support the brand.

Another way of saying the same thing is this: Brands are how businesses tell customers what to expect. When you fly on Southwest Airlines, you expect a cheap fare and to have fun. When you ship a package with FedEx, you expect it to get there in good shape and on time. When people come to our offices, they expect to pay a fair amount of money to have their lives changed with the best dentistry.

Brands Are Familiar Bridges

Brands are the familiar bridges across which people conduct business. At one end of your brand bridge is your office and you; at the other end are your patients. The bridge is the connection that takes the form of a very special kind of relationship—a relationship involving the kind of trust that only happens when two groups of people believe there is a direct connection between their value systems. We value "being the best" and "changing people's lives." Our patients are attracted to us because they value "having the best" and "having their lives changed." Now a brand bridge connects us. We have a values-based relationship. We trust each other. And when trust is present, decision-making is easy.

We never push people to accept treatment. We don't have to. Most of the time, they ask us whether we can do their dentistry. Now, all we do is say, "Yes." How sweet is that? Our higher-than-average fees rarely get in the way. This may sound strange to you, but our fee structure actually supports our brands because our patients expect to pay higher fees. In fact, if we didn't charge higher-than-average fees, the trust between our patients and us would be *weakened.*

Strong Personal Brands Are Distinctive, Relevant, and Consistent

David McNally and Karl Speak, authors of the book *Be Your Own Brand*, teach that strong personal brands have three characteristics: they're distinctive, relevant, and consistent.

Distinctive

Strong brands stand for something. They have a point of view. Your brand becomes strong when you decide what you believe in and commit yourself to acting on those beliefs. Standing up for your beliefs is often a courageous act. Courage of this kind is uncommon today. Thus, strong brands are distinctive.

Branding isn't image building. It isn't selling yourself to others. It results from understanding the needs of others, wanting to meet those needs, and being able to do so while being true to your values. Your values are the beliefs you hold true and the principles by which you live your life. Your brand is based on your values, not the other way around.

Relevant

Strong brands are relevant because what the brand stands for connects with what someone else considers important. We're successful only because there are many people in our areas who share our values. We earn relevance by the importance others place on *what* we do for them and by their judgment of *how* well we do it.

Consistent

Strong brands are consistent. Earlier you learned that brands tell customers what to expect. If customers don't get what they expect, the bridge connecting them and you is weakened. Consistency is the hallmark of all strong brands. FedEx is consistent in what it does. Tiger Woods is consistent in the messages he sends. We're consistent in the messages we convey to our communities.

Matt and Art's Personal Brand

Here is a statement of our personal brand: "We're the best restorative and cosmetic dentist in our areas. We change people's lives by changing their smiles." Our actions consistently exemplify our brand. The quality of our dentistry represents our brand. Our advertising portrays our brand. Many people have heard reports that enthusiastically support our brand from family, friends, and co-workers. Our brand is zapped into the minds of thousands of people in our areas. If we share common values across our personal brand bridge, then usually people come to see us. We treat them in ways that are consistent with the brand. They ask for the dentistry we love doing. They willingly pay our higher-than-average fees. We provide high-quality restorative and cosmetic dentistry that changes their lives. They tell their family and friends, who have similar values and who have also seen our advertisements. And the whole cycle begins again. Talk about being on a roll.

The $64,000 Question

So here's the $64,000 question: "What's your personal brand?" Write a two-sentence statement that describes it on the lines that follow:

_____

_____

_____

_____

_____

_____

How did it go? Did your personal brand statement include something about being the best dentist of your type in the area? If not, let that be your wake-up call to go get the training and then begin providing the care that will change your identity and your brand.

Your other choice is to remain average with an average brand doing average dentistry on average people while earning an average living. Not too exciting is it? The perpetuation of the average benefits no one—not your patients, not you, not our great profession.

Stop reading this chapter now unless you firmly hold some form of Empowering Belief #3:

I'm the best dentist in the area.

If you don't have Empowering Belief #3 firmly planted in your mind, the following information will be absolutely useless to you because the actions presented won't match your beliefs.

If you don't hold Empowering Belief #3 and choose to change it now, return to the chapter on How to Transform Your Beliefs and follow the instructions.

If you do believe "I'm the best dentist in the area," read on.

Actions That Exemplify Empowering Belief #3

You believe you're the best dentist of your type in the area. Congratulations. You've just put yourself on the hot seat. We're telling you this from personal experience. See, if your actions in the real world don't match the identity in your mind, you're going to get a "something is wrong" feeling in the pit of your stomach. This feeling will be your wake-up call to take action so your identity will again match your actions.

This wake-up call comes in two forms:

1. For some reason, the quality of the dental care you provide slips. You look at it and say, "This isn't like me. This isn't dentistry the best dentist in the area would do." The pain feels like a punch in the gut, and you take action to get your butt back on track.

2. You talk to someone or attend a dental presentation and see someone who is providing better care than you. You then feel compelled to learn what that person is doing so

you can maintain your identity as the best dentist in the area.

Here's something else to think about. The quality of your clinical, practice management, and relationship skills doesn't just hold steady. It's either improving or regressing. To stay the best and maintain the consistency of your brand, you will want to subscribe to a constant and never-ending improvement of your skills.

Here are nine actions that exemplify Empowering Belief #3:

1. Continue to learn the clinical, practice management, and relationship skills that will maintain your identity and support your personal brand as the best dentist in the area.

2. Make sure you hire people to work with you who are the best. Good is not good enough if you want to be the best.

3. Give your team members the training they need to be the best. Whenever we go to a training program, our teams come with us.

4. Buy the best equipment. Have the best facility. Use the best labs. There are many pieces in the "being the best" puzzle. Have them all in place.

5. Charge what you're worth. The old saying, "If you don't charge what you're worth, you will become worth what you charge," is absolutely true. Our fees are at least double the average fees in our area. And we're worth every penny of it.

6. Be the best in *and* out of the office. If you're the best, you need to be the best all the time. People are watching, looking for any chinks in your armor. This goes for your team, too.

7. If you're the best dentist in the area, effectively and consistently tell the people in your area the news. We will discuss how to do it in the chapter on Empowering Belief # 5: People Need to Know What We Do and How We Do It.

8. Be a role model for other dentists. In and out of the office be a person worthy of admiration.

9. Teach other dentists what you've learned and/or encourage them to attend the training programs you've used to become the best.

Conclusion

When you decide to be the best dentist in the area, almost everything will change. You will make major behavioral, structural, and practice management improvements in your office. If the transition from where you are now to where you want to go is smooth and orderly, chances are you're not making the transition at all. You're just rearranging the furniture. Once you move beyond rearranging the furniture and decide to throw almost all the old furniture out, you will have taken the first big step toward becoming the best dentist in your area.

So, to establish a new identity and create a new personal brand, you will need to take different actions. What a coincidence. That's the topic of the next chapter.

7

Empowering Belief #4:
To Have Different, I Must Do Different

In the Introduction, Matt told the story of how he met David Philip at LVI. At one time, David had a very successful dental practice according to conventional thinking. He was earning a good living doing good dentistry on lots of people. David had bought into two extremely damaging unwritten rules all dentists are taught. The two unwritten rules David adopted were:

1. Busy is better.
2. When you get busy, you add.

So, add he did—more patients, more treatment rooms, more team members, and more hours. Then David experienced extreme pain in the form of his son dying in a car accident and his own severe heart attack. David was smart. He paid attention to the signals life was sending him. If he hadn't, he would have experienced more pain for a much longer period of time.

Like the ghosts who visited Scrooge on Christmas Eve, David's two painful experiences got him thinking about what he truly valued in life. And being busy at the office certainly wasn't one of them. David decided he wanted to *have* extensive time with his family and to *have* a sense of professional fulfillment that comes with doing his favorite types of dentistry. With his desired *haves* firmly established, David chose to *do* the following:

- lighten the schedule and see fewer patients per day
- decrease the number of treatment rooms he used
- have fewer team members
- work fewer hours per day and fewer days per year
- stop doing dentistry he didn't enjoy and start doing more of the dentistry he enjoys
- raise his fees.

The actions he took achieved the *haves* David desired. As expected, he had more time with his family, and he had a renewed sense of professional fulfillment. Three unexpected *haves* also occurred:

1. The quality of his dentistry dramatically improved.
2. He made *more* money.
3. He enjoyed life more in and out of the office.

David Philip broke two unwritten rules and regained a life. He learned that less is more. He learned that to *have* different, he needed to *do* different. We all need to learn the same lessons.

What Do You Want?

In the second-to-last chapter of this book, you will identify what you want to *have* in five major areas of your life and what you need to *do* to make that happen. This chapter will be a big picture look at creating your future.

In this chapter, we're going to take a close look at the individual pieces of the puzzle that create your office brand. Both chapters are about doing. The last chapter is about doing the big things in your life. This chapter is about doing the smaller things in your practice.

On-Brand or Off-Brand?

In the last chapter, you learned that your brand is:

- an extension of who you are (your identity) and what you value
- a set of words and emotions stored in other people's heads
- a statement of what the people in your area can expect when they see you
- a familiar bridge across which you conduct business with your patients.

Our brand revolves around the words "the best," "life-changing," and "more expensive." We know every action we take must support our brand or the brand will be severely weakened by inconsistency. So we are constantly evaluating whether our actions, systems, and environments are on-brand (support our brand) or off-brand (don't support our brand). Here's an example of what we're talking about. In our offices, is wearing scrubs on-brand or off-brand? It's definitely off-brand. That's why we wear the clothing shown in the photos on the next page, which is on-brand.

It's not that wearing scrubs is good or bad. In oral surgery offices, the wearing of scrubs by the clinical part of the team would be on-brand. In an oral surgery office it would be on-brand for the front desk people to wear business attire.

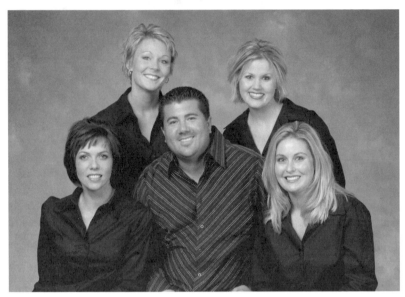

Matt's team

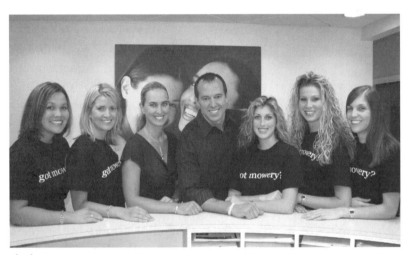

Art's team

Flip back to our office photos in the Introduction. Are the office exteriors and interiors on-brand or off-brand? We believe they're on-brand. Being on-brand is vitally important because it's not only *what* we do that's important. It's also *how* we do it. Providing high-quality dental care is *what* we do. Treating people fantastically and creating a wonderful office environment is *how* we do it. And if you want to establish a strong brand that attracts the people you want to see, "how you do it" must be on-brand.

Practice Separation

To create a memorable office brand, many or most of the on-brand actions you take will have to be different from what other offices in your area have done. This is great because it creates practice separation, which is *exactly* what you want. You don't want to be like everyone else. You're a group of people with unique identities. You have a brand that resonates with similar people. The last thing you want is to be like everybody else.

One of the most successful strategies for running our businesses is to check out what the other dentists in our areas are doing…*and do the exact opposite*. Here are some examples:

- They accept assignment of insurance. We don't.
- Many of them don't advertise at all because they believe it's unprofessional. We advertise all over the place.
- If they do advertise here, we advertise there.
- They have dozens of different fees for the restorations they do. We have two fees—one for direct restorations and one for indirect restorations.
- They act formally and professionally. We have a blast in the office and include our patients in the fun.
- They have their staff and patients call them doctor. We have our team and patients call us Matt and Art.

The Commodity Trap

Most dentists aren't like us. They have a commodity mentality. They think and act like all the other dentists in their areas. It must be safer for them that way. It's certainly how the insurance companies want dentists to think and act. That way they have more control over their herd.

But if you're a commodity, where's your identity and unique brand? And who in your area is going to be attracted to you? Certainly not people who share your values, because they don't know what your values are. If you're a commodity, people will think you're just like all those other dentists and come to you for all the wrong reasons, such as, "You were on the insurance list" or "Your office was close to my home."

If you're just like everybody else, your fees will need to be just like everybody else's. Again, that's just what the insurance companies want. Once you're in the commodity trap, it's a challenge to escape. It can be done, however, with the right strategy. We show dentists how to do it all the time in our *Achieving Extreme Success* seminar series.

Helpless and Hopeless—The Dangerous Duo

If you believe what you *do* isn't going to make any difference in what you can *have*, you feel helpless. If you believe it's always going to be that way, you feel hopeless. It's sad to say, but many dentists feel helpless and hopeless. Maybe that's why almost 70 percent of them wouldn't choose dentistry as a profession if they had to do it over again.

Charles Dickens begins his novel *A Tale of Two Cities*, "It was the best of times, it was the worst of times, it was the age of wisdom, it was the age of foolishness…." For us, this is the best of times. It's the best of times because we have wisdom. It's not luck; it's wisdom—wisdom that we put into action.

That's why we wrote this book and created our *Achieving Extreme Success* seminar series—to share the wisdom with you. We know the wisdom and the actions that follow will help you see you're not helpless, and it's not hopeless. We know the wisdom will set you free.

Stop reading this chapter now unless you firmly hold some form of Empowering Belief #4:

To have different, I must do different.

If you don't have Empowering Belief #4 firmly planted in your mind, the following information will be absolutely useless to you because the actions presented won't match your beliefs.

If you don't hold Empowering Belief #4 and choose to change it now, return to the chapter on How to Transform Your Beliefs and follow the instructions.

If you do believe "to have different, I must be different," read on.

Actions That Exemplify Empowering Belief #4

With your office brand clearly in mind, take the following actions, which exemplify Empowering Belief #4: To have different, I must do different:

1. Individually, have every team member walk around the exterior of your building. Have them create lists of everything they experience that is off-brand. They should use all five senses—sight, sound, touch, taste, and smell. Then, if possible, take action to make everything on the lists on-brand.

2. Individually, have every team member walk around the interior of your office. Have them create lists of everything

they experience that is off-brand. They should use all five senses—sight, sound, touch, taste, and smell. Then, take action to make everything on the lists on-brand.

3. Individually, have each team member park his or her car where patients do, walk into the office, sit in the reception area, and go to the patient restroom. Have them make lists of everything they experience that is off-brand. They should use all five senses—sight, sound, touch, taste, and smell. Then, take action to make everything on the lists on-brand.

4. When team members do their recare visits, have them make lists of everything they experience that is off-brand. They should use all five senses—sight, sound, touch, taste, and smell. Then, take action to make everything on the lists on-brand.

5. When team members have restorations completed, have them make lists of everything they experience that is off-brand. They should use all five senses—sight, sound, touch, taste, and smell. Then, take action to make everything on the lists on-brand.

6. Individually, have each team member pretend to be a new patient and run through the same procedures a new patient would. Have all of them make lists of everything they experience that is off-brand. They should use all five senses—sight, sound, touch, taste, and smell. Then take action to make everything on the lists on-brand.

7. As a group, examine all your internal marketing, external marketing, and public relations actions. Identify everything that is off-brand. Then create a plan to make everything on the list on-brand.

8. As a group, examine all your interactions with patients. Identify everything you do that is off-brand. Then create a plan

to make the interactions totally on-brand. Examine the following interactions:

a. the first phone call
b. the time period between the first phone call and the first visit
c. the first visit
d. the time period between the first and second visit
e. the treatment conference
f. the time period between the treatment conference and the first clinical visit
g. perio therapy visits
h. restorative visits
i. recare visits
j. the time period between recare visits

9. Take a close look at how you present yourself to the community when you are out of the office. Is there anything you do that is off-brand? If the answer is "yes," think how can you make it on-brand. Remember, strong personal brands are consistent.

10. Take a close look at how the other people on your team present themselves to the community when they are out of the office. Have a group discussion on this topic and stress how important it is for them to be on-brand in public.

Conclusion

This chapter was about doing. And doing on-brand activities is by far the best way to establish your brand in the minds of the people in your community. It's not the only way, however. You can also let people know what you do and how you do it with marketing and public relations. Read on to see why this is so important.

8

Empowering Belief #5:

People Need to Know What We Do and How We Do It

In the last chapter, you learned why it's so important to free yourself from the boundaries established by unwritten rules. It's not your fault the unwritten rules are there. They were placed in your mind long ago by people who aren't practicing dentists. It's easy for them to sit back and pontificate about the way things should be. They aren't responsible for your payroll. They don't see your patients. They shouldn't tell you how to run your practice or live your life.

This chapter will be another unwritten rule-buster for you because it will take the "being different" and "practice separation" message one step further. You will learn that you must communicate to everyone in your area what you do and how you do it.

If they think about it at all, most dentists believe they deliver average-quality care. As a result, they charge average fees, use average labs, receive average training, have average equipment, hire average people, and earn about the same amount of money as most other dentists. They attend the average meetings so they can hang around a whole bunch of other average dentists. In addition, average dentists have no reason or desire to let people in their areas know what they do and how they do it. They just wait for average patients to choose them.

If you have an empowering belief that you're the best dentist in the area, you will automatically charge higher fees, use the best labs, receive lots of the best training, have the best equipment, hire the best people, and do the best dentistry. In addition, you will have no problem creating practice separation with the other offices in your area by repeatedly and effectively letting people know what you do and how you do it.

Playing It Safe

We both practice in very conservative areas of the country. When starting our practices, we mistakenly played it safe and did yellow pages advertising just like everybody else. That's what our unwritten rules directed us to do, and we didn't want to ruffle the feathers of the established dentists in our areas. The yellow pages ads worked okay, but they didn't attract the people who wanted the kinds of dentistry we wanted to do.

Plus, playing it safe just didn't feel right, which was a great way to discover that our actions weren't matching our identities. So we drastically changed the way we let people know what we do and how we do it. We firmly believe it was the right thing to do. If we didn't do it and do it well, hundreds of people in our communities would miss out on *receiving* the very best that dentistry has to offer. And that would be a crying shame. In addition, we would miss out on *providing* the very best that dentistry has to offer. That's a lose/lose situation. We're into win/win. We hope you are, too.

Look around at the people in the world who are extraordinary. They don't play it safe. Donald Trump doesn't play it safe when he makes a deal to build an office building. Steven Jobs didn't play it safe when he went up against the big boys with his iPods, iTunes, and iPhones. Oprah Winfrey doesn't play it safe with her TV program, production company, magazine, movies, and Broadway shows. Playing it safe is habit forming and leads to a life of mediocrity. How exciting is that?

> *"You're only given a little spark of madness.*
> *You mustn't lose it."*
>
> **—Robin Williams**

Stop reading this chapter now unless you firmly hold Empowering Belief #5:

People need to know what we do and how we do it.

If you don't have Empowering Belief #5 firmly planted in your mind, the following information will be absolutely useless to you because the actions presented won't match your beliefs.

If you don't hold Empowering Belief #5 and choose to change it now, return to the chapter on How to Change Your Beliefs and follow the instructions.

If you do believe that "people need to know what we do and how we do it," read on.

Actions That Exemplify and Reinforce Empowering Belief #5

Stuart Britt once said, "Doing business without advertising is like winking at a girl in the dark. You know what you're doing, but nobody else does."

Stuart was right. You can be the best dentist in the area, but if people don't know about it, nobody wins. There are three ways to let people know what you do and how you do it—internal marketing, external marketing, and public relations. It's vital that you use a nice mix of the three because brand strength comes from repeated impressions.

Internal Marketing

Internal marketing is the process of marketing to the patients you already have and working with your current patients to attract new ones. Internal marketing has the advantages of being extremely effective when done properly and very low cost.

External Marketing

External marketing includes phone book ads, newspaper and magazine print ads, direct mail, Internet marketing, radio and TV commercials, and alternative advertising such as airport signs and billboards. Most dentists don't do much, if any, external marketing. It's taboo for them because they're so worried about what the other dentists in town will say. What are the other dentists so afraid of? Their favorite phrase is, "Advertising in *not* professional." This is just another way of saying, "We don't want anyone to stand out from the crowd. We want everyone to be part of the herd."

> "Collective fear stimulates the herd instinct, and tends to produce ferocity toward those who are not regarded as members of the herd."
>
> **—Bertrand Russell**

We don't have a problem breaking away from the herd and marketing aggressively. Why should we? We're the best at what we do, and everyone in our areas should know it. Our external marketing plans include all of the methods mentioned above.

We don't want to tell you what to do because an effective external marketing plan varies depending on your office brand and the competition in the marketplace. What works for us may not work for you.

The amount of money we spend each month on external marketing varies. We both invest about ten percent of our yearly grosses in external marketing.

Public Relations

The definition of public relations is the business of inducing the public to have understanding for and goodwill toward a person or business. Public relations is not traditional external marketing. With public relations, you don't pay a newspaper to place an ad. You make it easy for them to write an article about you. You can hire an external public relations person, or you can have an interested person in your office be the PR person.

We always stay in the public eye by attending and supporting various charity events. We also do many pro bono cases for deserving members of our community. We don't advertise our generosity, but someone in the media almost always catches wind of it.

Create an Attractive Website That Shows People What You Do and How You Do It

When it comes to high-end reconstructive and cosmetic dentistry, the Web is the yellow pages of the 21st century. As a result, it's vital that you have an attractive website. It needs to be attractive in two ways:

1. The appearance of your website must be first rate. It should have numerous "before-and-after" photos of cases you've completed.

2. The website must be a magnet for people who enter words such as "cosmetic dentistry" into search engines such as Google. When people enter the words "cosmetic dentistry (your city)," where on the list does your office website appear? It should be at the top of the first page. If not, you have some work to do.

> "If you want to be found, stand where the seeker seeks."
>
> **—Sidney Lanier**

Conclusion

After doing a fantastic job of letting people in your area know what you do and how you do it, some of them will come to your office. It's vital that you have a team of people who can form close relationships, provide on-brand service, and help them receive the care they desire and deserve. Read on to discover how to build an outstanding team.

In our two-day Achieving Extreme Success seminar series, we always present the newest and best ways we're promoting our practices with internal and external marketing and public relations.

To learn more about our Achieving Extreme Success seminar series and our other products and services, go to www.BynumMoweryWay.com.

9

Empowering Belief #6:
Staff Is an Infection, Team Is the Cure

This may be the most important chapter in the whole book. We say this because we've seen firsthand the rapid improvements that are made rapidly when a dental staff becomes HOT—a High-Octane Team. Let's examine the difference between a staff person and a team player and how a collection of team players creates a High-Octane Team.

Staff Person

When it comes to any organization, what characteristics pop into your mind when you hear the words "staff person"? You may think of people who:

- have a job.
- are told what to do.
- do their duties and not much more. Their favorite phrase is, "That's not my job."
- punch a time clock and work a set number of hours.
- do average-quality work.
- pass their staff infection on to other members of the staff.
- work for "the man."

- constantly think "me, me, me."
- are employed by an average company that produces average results.

Webster's Dictionary defines staff as "the personnel who assist a director in carrying out an assigned task." What a bunch of bull! Just hearing that definition makes us want to barf. How inspiring would it be for you to "assist a director in carrying out an assigned task"? Not very, we're guessing.

Yet, most dentists are directors who have staffs. That's how it's always been done. That's the safe, highly-regimented, predictable way. That's the unwritten rule. We believe the unwritten rule sucks. We believe staff is an infection, and team is the cure.

Team Player

What characteristics pop into your mind when you hear the words "team player?" You may think of people who:

- have a position.
- make important decisions after being well trained.
- do whatever it takes to get the job done. Their favorite phrase is, "How can I help?"
- are willing to come early or stay late to go the extra mile.
- do their best work.
- pass their team-player mentality on to other members of the team.
- work with the team and the clients.
- constantly think, "we, we, we."
- work with an exceptional company that produces exceptional results.

The High-Octane Team

Let's move from individuals to groups. Think of the worst group you've been part of. This could be a sports, work, or volunteer organization group. What three factors made it so bad? Does your list of factors include no commonly accepted goal, poor leadership, lack of talent, and people not supporting others while personally doing the bare minimum? Sounds like a staff infection to us.

Now, think of the best group you were ever part of. What factors made it such an outstanding group? Did your list of factors include a commonly accepted goal, effective leadership, abundant talent, and people gladly supporting others while personally going above-and-beyond? Sounds like a High-Octane Team to us.

To create a High-Octane Team, you need to take a leap of faith—which is another way of saying you need to change a cherished belief. You need to stop being a director who assigns tasks and demands they be completed and become a player-coach* who hires the right people, gives them the necessary training, and then *steps back and allows* the team members the freedom to do their jobs.

We highlighted the words *steps back and allows* in the previous sentence because that is the most difficult part of the team-building process. It's ironic that you have to "let go" in order to have more happiness and success in your practice. Most dentists' success strategy is to "hang on tighter." As a result, they have less. We "let go" and have more. We "let go" because we firmly believe that staff is an infection and team is the cure. We hope you do, too.

*In the early years of the National Basketball Association (NBA), there were player-coaches—people who both played in the games and coached the team.

Stop reading this chapter now unless you firmly hold Empowering Belief #6:

Staff is an infection, team is the cure.

If you don't have Empowering Belief #6 firmly planted in your mind, the following information will be absolutely useless to you because the actions presented won't match your beliefs.

If you don't hold Empowering Belief #6 and choose to change it now, return to the chapter on How to Change Your Beliefs and follow the instructions.

If you do believe that "staff is an infection and team is the cure," read on.

Actions That Exemplify and Reinforce Empowering Belief #6

Henry Ford said, "Teamwork is the ability to work together toward a common vision. The ability to direct individual accomplishments toward organizational objectives. It is the fuel that allows common people to attain uncommon results."

We agree. The uncommon results we've achieved in our practices are primarily due to our ability to create and maintain awesome teams. Believe it or not, it's simple to do, as the following six ways will show you. But just because it's simple doesn't mean it's easy. It will require you to hold fast to your team mentality and help others do the same. It will consistently require you to step outside your comfort zone. The rewards, however, will be worth it!

Six Ways to Create a High-Octane Team

1. Beginning today, replace the word "staff" with the word "team" when you speak and write. This may seem like a small act, but words and emotions are the building blocks of belief. When you say the word "team," you add a tiny thread to the team concept rope in your mind. After you add enough tiny threads, the rope becomes stronger and finally unbreakable.

   If you say or write the word "staff," immediately substitute the word "team." If you say the word "staff" at the office, put $10 in a jar to be used for a "team" party later on. If a team member says the word "staff," he or she should add $1.

2. Hire for attitude and train for skill. The following fable illustrates what we mean:

   > A traveler met a sage on the road to a city. He asked, "What are the people like in the city ahead?"
   >
   > The sage answered, "What were the people like in the city from which you came?"
   >
   > The traveler replied, "Lazy, untrustworthy, and stupid. I couldn't wait to leave."
   >
   > "Ah," said the sage, "then you will find them the same in the city ahead."
   >
   > Shortly afterward, a second traveler approached the sage and asked the same question, "What are the people like in the city ahead?"
   >
   > Again the sage answered, "What were the people like in the city from which you came?"
   >
   > The second traveler replied, "Honest, hard-working, and friendly. I was sorry I had to leave."
   >
   > "Ah," repeated the sage, "then you will find them the same in the city ahead."

This fable illustrates a fundamental truth about human behavior: People have varying degrees of positive and negative attitudes. Attitudes are nothing more than a collection of beliefs about self, the world, and the people in it. They interpret their world through these attitudes and get out of life what they look for.

This is why it's vital to hire team members with great attitudes. Select people you would enjoy hanging with outside the office. At interviews, watch out for people who interrupt when you're talking. We've learned this is a really bad sign. If your gut tells you something's wrong with the person, go with your feeling.

People can easily fake having a positive attitude during a thirty-minute interview in your office. To get around this, have the person go to lunch with your team (minus you) away from the office. If the team decides the person has potential, schedule a one-week, paid working interview.

It's wonderful if the person you bring into the team also has the necessary skills to do the job effectively. If they don't have the skills, their positive attitude will propel them to learn what they need to know.

3. Add the phrase "and whatever it takes to give on-brand service to all our patients" to the end of everyone's job descriptions. Stress the "whatever it takes" concept to your team. Make it a big deal!

4. Recognize and reward the team-oriented actions you want to see more of. Any time team members do something you would like to see repeated, immediately reinforce the actions with praise or a compliment. When the entire team goes the extra mile, do something fun and unexpected as a group.

5. Collect stories of team members who have given on-brand service and tell the stories often to your team, your patients, and your community.

> "The best leaders…almost without exception and at every level, are master users of stories and symbols."
>
> **—Tom Peters**

6. The most effective way to create an awesome team is to install a system in which every team member shares in the success of the practice. There are several different ways this can be done. In our *Achieving Extreme Success* seminar series, we teach two very effective systems. A word of caution here: The entire team must be on board to implement any system you choose, and the system must be implemented properly.

Conclusion

Believing that staff is an infection and team is the cure is a vitally important empowering belief for you to adopt. Like a boomerang, it will return to create a successful dental practice and an abundant life.

There is another empowering belief that takes this team concept to a higher level. That belief is Empowering Belief #7: I'm here to serve my team and patients. Luckily, that's the subject of the next chapter.

10

Empowering Belief #7:
I'm Here to Serve My Team and Patients

A famous singer was scheduled to appear at a Paris opera house. Ticket sales boomed, and the night of the concert found the house full and every ticket sold.

A feeling of anticipation and excitement was in the air as the house manager stepped out on the stage and announced, "Ladies and gentlemen, thank you for your enthusiastic support, but I have news that may be disappointing to some. An accident, not serious in nature but serious enough, will prevent the woman you have come to hear from performing tonight." He went on to give the name of the understudy who would step into the role, but the crowd groaned and drowned it out. The excitement in the audience turned to bitter disappointment and frustration as the opera began.

The stand-in artist gave the performance everything she had. Throughout the evening, there had been nothing but an uneasy silence. Even at the end, no one applauded.

Then from the balcony, the thin voice of a little boy broke the silence. "Mommy," he called out, "I think you were wonderful!" The crowd was silent for a second and then broke into thunderous applause.

In many ways, your dental office is like the opera house. The team members are the understudies, and you are the little boy in the balcony. When you praise your team after they've given their performances everything they have, they will feel fantastic, do even better the next time, and enjoy walking in the door every day. And if they're happy, there's a really good chance you're going to be happy.

Team Comes First, Patients Come Second

There are two groups of people who walk into your office each day: your patients and your team. Which one is more important? It's very easy to get totally preoccupied with serving your patients because there's a sense of urgency associated with them. ("We need to take great care of them now because they're here for only a short period of time, and they pay the bills.") But we believe your team is more important even though there isn't that same sense of urgency associated with them. ("They're here all the time, and they don't pay the bills.")

A great way to gauge whether you put your team first is to examine your actions after a patient complains about a team member. Do you automatically think, "The patient is right," then call the person to apologize for the team member's poor behavior? Southwest Airlines legendary CEO, Herb Kelleher, wouldn't do something like that. When asked whether the customer is always right, Kelleher answered, "No, they're not! And I think that's one of the biggest betrayals of employees a boss can possibly commit. The customer is sometimes wrong. We don't carry those sorts of customers. We write them and say, 'Fly somebody else. Don't abuse our people.'"

Southwest's president, Colleen Barrett, agrees with Herb when she says, "We're in the customer service business. We happen to offer air transportation. We consider our employees to be our number-one customer. Our passengers are second, and our shareholders are third. As leaders, if we give great customer service to our employees, they will in turn provide it to their customers who are the passengers. And the rewards will be there for our shareholders."

Not only is Kelleher's and Barrett's way "the right thing to do," but also how do you think the Southwest Airlines team reacts when they hear their bosses went to bat for them? They respond with a truckload of loyalty no paycheck will ever buy.

Like Southwest Airlines, when you put your team first and patients second, you will *increase* the level of service to the patients, not decrease it. When you treat your team with more care and concern, they will treat your patients with more care and concern. Your patients will then accept more comprehensive dentistry. Everybody wins when you put your team first.

"Life is a place of service.

Joy can be real only if people look upon their life

as a service and have a definite object in life

outside themselves and their personal happiness."

—Leo Tolstoy

Invert the Pyramid

The organizational pyramid for most dental offices looks like Figure A shown here.

At the top of the pyramid is the doctor. The doctor is the supreme commander of the entire dental operation. Everyone else is beneath, so the doctor has to be looked up

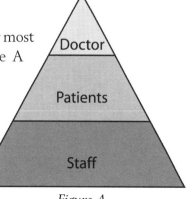

Figure A

to. The patients are the next level down. They are treated by the doctor, who tells them what dental care they need. The lowly staff is on the bottom of the pyramid because it's their job to serve the patients and the doctor.

We believe the pyramid should be inverted as shown in Figure B below. The team should come first and be on top, where they belong. The patients come second, and the doctor is at the bottom. The doctor is still the leader, but a servant leader.

Figure B

Inverting your office pyramid and becoming a servant leader may be two of the most challenging things you will ever do in your professional career—and the most vitally important. It will require dropping a massive load of your ego. We used the word "load" in the previous sentence on purpose. It feels heavy being alone at the top. Sure, you're the boss, but that gets old in a hurry. It's tiring constantly telling people what to do, demanding that they do it, and correcting them when they don't.

We know this from our experience. At one time in our careers, both of us arranged our offices according to Figure A. It was an unwritten rule we bought into. We got tired of feeling heavy, so we changed. Now we feel light and take things lightly. Our team, patients, and families feel it. We encourage you to lighten up, too.

> "Mountains appear more lofty the nearer they are approached, but great leaders resemble them not in this particular."
>
> **—Marguerite Blessington**

Culture—The Invisible Framework

Servant leaders also pay close attention to the cultures of their organizations. Culture is the invisible framework that supports and gives justification to the actions of the entire team. The individual pieces of that framework are the team's values. Values are deep-seated beliefs about the world and how it operates. Values are also the guidelines people use to make decisions. Walt Disney's brother, Roy, summed it up best when he said, "When values are clear, decisions are easy."

Maintaining a culture and instilling values isn't easy. Organizations have to work at it consistently. One reason Southwest Airlines has been so successful over its history is because of the culture Southwest has created and maintained. Herb Kelleher says, "Culture is the most precious thing a company has, so you must work harder at it than anything else."

The Walt Disney Company agrees. Every new employee, whether it's a senior vice president or a person sweeping the sidewalks at a Disney theme park, must take a two-day Disney traditions training program. Through a history lesson on the origins of the Disney tradition and stories of people who have exemplified its values, each person learns what it means to represent The Walt Disney Company. When finished, their actions are purposeful and their decision-making process is clear.

So how do you create and maintain an outstanding culture in your dental office? It's deceptively simple. *Decide what's important and talk about it over and over.* We believe it's important to change people's lives, to give patients on-brand service, to offer them the best that dentistry has to offer, to have fun, to earn a great living, *and* to have lots of time with our families. So we talk about all these things over and over.

> **Stop reading this chapter now unless you firmly hold Empowering Belief #7:**
>
> **I'm here to serve my team and patients.**
>
> If you don't have Empowering Belief #7 firmly planted in your mind, the following information will be absolutely useless to you because the actions presented won't match your beliefs.
>
> If you don't hold Empowering Belief #7 and choose to change it now, return to the chapter on How to Change Your Beliefs and follow the instructions.
>
> If you do believe "I'm here to serve my team and patients," read on.

Actions That Exemplify and Reinforce Empowering Belief #7

Here are five actions that exemplify Empowering Belief #7: I'm here to serve my team and patients:

1. Make a copy of the Figure B pyramid. Then put it somewhere you will see it every day you're in the office to remind you to be a servant leader.

2. When a patient complains to you about a team member and it's obvious the patient is in the wrong, support your team member. Then, let the patient know how you feel and make it clear you won't tolerate that kind of behavior in the future. Maybe offer him or her the option of seeing someone else. Make sure your team members hear how you have supported them.

3. Use Art's "Fire Five Rule." Next week, hold a team meeting and choose five patients you're going to fire. These are the people whom everyone dislikes to see on the schedule and

whose actions tie your intestines into little knots. Call them and explain why your relationship just isn't working out.

4. Decide what's important in your office and talk about it over and over.

5. Use the four words "How can I help?" repeatedly. These words are magical as they automatically invert your pyramid. Say them frequently to your team and patients.

Team Examples

- "Angie, I know you want to be at you daughter's soccer game at 5 P.M. How can I help you get out right at 4:30?"

- "Tammy, our new magazine ad is really generating a lot of phone calls. How can I help you handle them all well?"

- "Snow, how can I help you stay up-to-date on all the new advances in perio therapy?"

Patient Examples

- "Lindsey, thanks for coming into our office today. How can I help?"

- "Kelly, I know you want to have those veneers done. How can I help you have them?"

- "Mickey, we've just talked about good dentistry, better dentistry, and the best dentistry you can have. We're here to serve you. What's the best way we can help?"

Conclusion

The walls of Southwest Airlines corporate headquarters are filled with photos of passengers and team members. The idea was Colleen Barrett's. She wanted to make the sterile corporate walls more homelike. Barrett will retire in 2008. When asked what words she would like to see on a plaque under her photo after she goes, Barrett replied, "She cared."

After you retire, what words will they put on the plaque under your photo on the wall? Will it be "He fixed teeth," "She made a lot of money," or "He was the boss"? Or will it be "She cared," "She was a servant leader," or "He changed people's lives"? The choices you make from this moment on will determine the words on your plaque. Choose wisely and well.

The next chapter, I Must Make Emotional Connections with People, is an extension of this one. Colleen Barrett connects emotionally with her teammates because she cares. And people don't care how much you know until they know how much you care.

11

Empowering Belief #8:

I Must Make Emotional Connections with People

Dr. David Philip's little speech at LVI had logical and emotional components. The logical part got our attention. The emotional part moved us to action. It's the same with all your interactions with team members and patients in your office. There are logical and emotional components to the relationships, and it's the emotional parts that determine whether your office is ordinary or extraordinary.

Most dentists are way too logical. Logical people are the ones who tend to do well in pre-dental subjects. The DAT is purely logical. Our dental school training is almost 100 percent logical. The dental board examinations are logical, and almost all post-graduate training is on the logical side of dentistry.

And yet it's emotion that moves people to action. That's why the majority of dentists struggle with a profession that should be extremely fulfilling. They focus on logic and ignore emotion. Luckily, we can all learn ways to add a layer of emotion to all our interactions with team members and patients.

People Want Emotions

When it comes right down to it, people want emotions. They don't really want money. They want the emotions (success, security, or status) they believe money will give them. People don't want material possessions, relationships, or jobs. They want the emotions they believe those things will give them. Likewise, patients don't want dentistry. They want the emotions they believe the dental care will give them.

So here's our question to you: "How much attention do you pay to adding emotion to all your interactions with the people in your office?" If your answer is "Not much," read on as we explore the emotional topics of rapport, likeability, fun, and loyalty.

Rapport

The definition of rapport is "a relationship marked by harmony, accord, and affinity." Sounds like a pretty good way to do business in a dental office. Our language gives away the essence of rapport. When we have rapport with someone, we say things like, "We're on the same wavelength" or "We're in sync."

Rapport is vital for any deep and lasting relationship. The secret to gaining rapport can be found in the definition of the French word from which it is derived. The French word is "*raporter*," meaning "to give back." When two people are in rapport, they continually give back to each in the form of:

- nodding in agreement
- returning a smile
- empathizing with a problem
- matching energy levels
- discussing commonalities.

After a while, they're on the same wavelength and in sync.

Likeability

Likeability is purely emotional. Tim Adams, the author of the outstanding book *The Likeability Factor*, defines likeability as "the ability to create positive attitudes in other people through the delivery of emotional and physical benefits." We believe likeability is the overlooked secret to success. Think about it: There are hundreds of personal success books written each year. Most of them focus on the choices people must make in their daily lives to be successful. These books ignore one simple truth: *Your success in life is heavily influenced by other people's choices concerning you.*

Isn't success in your professional life determined by who wants to be part of your team, who wants to come to your practice, and how often they decide to proceed with comprehensive care? Isn't success in your personal life determined by who wants to hang with you or have a romantic relationship with you? Think about the person who cuts your hair. Do you like the person? Based on the thousands of people to whom we've asked that question, there's a 95 percent chance that you *do* like the person. People do business with people they like.

If you doubt the importance of likeability, consider the following:

In a study done in 1992 at the University of Toronto, Dr. Phillip Noll surveyed fifty divorced and fifty married couples. He found that people who scored high on a likeability evaluation had divorce rates 50 percent lower than the general population. If both partners were likeable, the divorce rate was reduced another 50 percent.

Several studies have shown that likeable patients receive better medical care. A St. James University Hospital study, conducted in Leeds, England, showed that children with likeable parents received better healthcare, longer appointments, and more follow-up visits. A University of California study conducted by Barbara Gerbert revealed that likeable patients were encouraged to call their physicians and return for care more frequently.

Alice Burkin, a leading medical malpractice lawyer, says, "People just don't sue doctors they like." Research done by Wendy Levinson confirms Burkin's statement. As described in *Blink: The Power of Thinking without Thinking* by Malcolm Gladwell, Levinson recorded hundreds of doctor-patient conversations. She then divided the doctors into two groups: those who had never been sued and those who had been sued at least twice. She found that the doctors who had never been sued (1) spent more than three minutes longer with their patients, (2) were more likely to engage in active listening by making statements such as, "Go on, tell me more about that," and (3) were far more likely to laugh or be funny during the visit. There was no difference in the amount or quality of the information they gave their patients concerning the patient's condition or details about medication. The difference between the doctors who were sued and those who weren't was entirely in *how* they talked to their patients (emotion), not *what* they said (logic).

Fun

Those of you who know us personally realize we have fun in most everything we do. We have fun at the office. We walk in with smiles. We walk out with bigger smiles. We have fun at home with our wives and kids. We have fun at our *Achieving Extreme Success* seminar series. Most dental seminars are so boring it's pathetic.

Southwest Airlines knows about having fun. Their hilarious hijinks are legendary. On one Southwest Airlines flight, a man opened the overhead compartment to put his briefcase in. As he did, a flight attendant stuck her head out and shouted, "BOOOOO!" She was hiding in the overhead compartment. We haven't seen that on Delta in a while. The whole planeload of people cracked up, and we proceeded to have a wonderful trip.

On another flight, a man with a broken leg, crutches, and a huge cast was walking down the jet way. A flight attendant stopped him at the door, pointed at his leg, and said, "Looks like you've been flying America West."

Southwest Airlines knows there are three bottom-line benefits to having fun:

1. *More productivity.* Southwest Airlines has the smallest number of employees per aircraft, serves the most customers per employee, and has the most enviable record of profitability in the industry.

2. *Lower attrition and absenteeism.* People who are enjoying their day are more apt to stick with a company/practice and come to work every day. Southwest's attrition rate and absenteeism are believed to be the lowest in the airline industry.

3. *Customers respond more positively.* Southwest has less than half the complaints per passenger than the No. 2 airline.

> "If I can get you to laugh with me, you like me better, which makes you more open to my ideas."
>
> **—John Cleese**

If you can't have fun in dentistry and make it fun for your team and patients, change what you're doing or get out of the profession. Life's too short not to.

Case Acceptance

We could write a whole book (and we may) on how emotional connections influence case acceptance. Most dentists attempt to convince people logically to accept treatment plans. Their approach can be summed up as, "I'm the expert. Here are your problems. Here's what I think you should do." It's no wonder they're frustrated and have such low case acceptance rates.

Our care acceptance approach is almost totally emotional. Sometimes, with our cosmetic patients, we even shed a tear together when we discuss the pain they've experienced in the past and/or when they see their new smiles for the first time.

We attract patients who have the same values we have and gain rapport with them. We come to trust and like each other. We understand them by learning their unique stories, and they understand the quality of care we deliver. We care about their well-being. Only then do we offer three choices of care (good, better, best) and say, "We're here to serve you. What's the best way we can help?"

We know that sounds simple, and it is. But it's not easy to do consistently. It takes the right patients interacting with the right team members who have the right attitudes and do the right things.

> "People like people like themselves.
> People trust people like themselves.
> People buy from people they trust."

Loyalty

If a $50,000 piece of equipment were missing from your dental office tomorrow morning, how concerned would you be? How hard would you work to recover it? What steps would you take to make sure it didn't happen again? I'm betting you would be tremendously concerned; you wouldn't stop looking until you got it back; and you would make darn sure it didn't happen again.

We have a very important question for you: "Would you take the same steps if you lost a loyal patient or one valued team member?" We hope so, because their value is considerably higher than $50,000.

We've never seen the figures for dental practices, but the average U.S. corporation loses half its customers every five years, half its employees every four years, and half its investors every two years. What a waste. We do know this: Patient and team member loyalty can be the difference between you having a moderately or wildly successful dental practice.

Most dental practices have satisfied patients. We have loyal patients. There's a huge difference. Satisfied patients are fine, but they don't create positive word-of-mouth advertising, refer numerous other people, or easily accept comprehensive care like loyal patients do.

Most dentists have a satisfied staff. We have a loyal team. It's a huge advantage for us because our loyal team members do their best work, go above-and-beyond, and will be there with us through thick and thin.

You can create satisfaction logically, but you can't create loyalty logically. You create loyalty emotionally by loving people. Love isn't talked about enough in dentistry. Funny, the folks at Southwest Airlines talk about it all the time. Their ticker symbol is LUV.

Not only does love make life worth living, but it's also a key component of achieving extreme success in your dental practice. Look up the word "love" in the dictionary. The definition is "deeply understanding and caring about another person." Do you understand and care for your teammates and patients? Or do you just tolerate them? Your answers to those two questions will determine the amount of professional fulfillment you experience and the amount of financial success you achieve…because it's the emotional connection with people that makes the difference.

Stop reading this chapter now unless you firmly hold Empowering Belief #8:

I must make emotional connections with people.

If you don't have Empowering Belief #8 firmly planted in your mind, the following information will be absolutely useless to you because the actions presented won't match your beliefs.

If you don't hold Empowering Belief #8 and choose to change it now, return to the chapter on How to Change Your Beliefs and follow the instructions.

If you do believe "I must make emotional connections with people," read on.

Actions That Exemplify and Reinforce Empowering Belief #8

Here are six actions that exemplify Empowering Belief #8: I must make emotional connections with people.

1. Have a complimentary "meet-and-greet" visit with your new patients. No doctor time needs to be scheduled. Just have a team member sit down with patients and get to know each other. Apply the "Seven-Minute Rule" to the conversation, which is "Don't talk teeth for the first seven minutes." Then, discover what they desire and share your office philosophy. Give the patients a tour of the office and introduce the team. Together, make the decision to meet again. If you

discover your office isn't the right place, thank them for thinking of you and refer them to an office that can better meet their needs.

2. Establish rapport with your new patients by getting on their wavelength. Sit down with them in a relaxed, non-clinical environment and shoot the breeze. Discover something you have in common with them and talk about that for a little bit. If they send you a message in an excited manner, give it back to them by being excited, too.

3. Be likeable by giving people sincere compliments, doing little, unexpected things for them, and thanking them for their friendship. Don't just talk about clinical topics. Discuss personal subjects at the beginning and end of each visit.

4. Make having fun a priority in your office. Once a month, at a team meeting, evaluate the things you can do to have more fun in the office. Take a look at the negative things you can eliminate or lessen and the positive things you can enhance. Remember, decide what's important and talk about it over and over.

5. Focus on patient loyalty, not patient satisfaction. At your weekly team meetings, ask the loyalty question: "How can we treat our patients so they are compelled to tell someone else how great we are?"

Conclusion

In his must-read book, *Lovemarks: The Future Beyond Brands,* Kevin Roberts writes, "The social fabric of North America is spread thinner than ever. People are looking for new, emotional connections. They're looking for products and services they can love. They are looking for more ways they can connect."

Your dental office can be a place where people find new, emotional connections, the place where people find the services they love, and the place where people deeply connect. What a special place that would be!

12

Empowering Belief #9:
I Dream Big in Everything I Do

What if you slept?

And what if,

in your sleep

you dreamed?

And what if,

in your dream,

you went to heaven

and there plucked

a strange and beautiful flower?

And what if,

when you awoke,

you had the flower in your hand?

—Samuel Taylor Coleridge

What If?

Coleridge used the words "what if" four times in his poem. We think he's on to something extremely powerful. The words "what if" immediately shift your thinking, don't they? The words mentally and magically transport you from where you are now to where you could be. They transform your aspirations into your possibilities. They tear down barriers and build a bridge from your current reality to your big dream.

Albert Einstein knew the power of "what if?" Einstein was the scientist who developed the theory that time stops when you travel at the speed of light. He didn't come up with such a revolutionary idea by feverishly working with his slide rule late at night. He got the idea while sitting at his kitchen table at noon. He looked up at a clock on the wall and asked a question that had never been asked before. He thought, "*What if* I could hop on a light wave that came off that clock at exactly twelve noon? As I ride on the light wave off into the distance at the speed of light with all the twelve o'clock light waves traveling alongside me, I wonder if time would stop no matter how far I went?" His answer was obviously "Yes!"

Like Albert Einstein, if you want different answers in your life, you need to ask different questions—questions that break down preconceived barriers and limiting paradigms— questions that transform your dreams into realities.

Jim Carrey Dreams Big

Jim Carrey was born on January 17, 1962, in Newmarket, Ontario. His mother, Kathleen, suffered from depression and was often chronically sick with real and imagined illnesses. In an earlier chapter, you learned about seven-year-old Jim having the thought, "I'm going to prove to my mother that I'm a miracle, and that her life is worth something."

His father, Percy, was a sharp-witted and highly amusing guy. As a young man, Percy played the saxophone in a big band. But Percy sold his sax and his dreams to take a job as an accountant. Jim never forgot what that dashed dream did to his dad.

As a child, Jim obsessively studied TV shows, perfecting his impressions of the stars. He loved putting on one-man shows for his family in the basement of their home. The Christmas season was the best time of year for Jim because visiting relatives increased the size of his audience.

In junior high school Jim insisted on performing for his classmates. The teachers soon realized the only way to calm him down was to allow ten minutes at the end of each school day for his performance. Believe it or not, Jim would occasionally wear tap shoes to bed in case his parents needed cheering up in the middle of the night.

When Jim was in the ninth grade, Percy lost his job, and the family was forced to sell its home. To make ends meet, the whole family took jobs as security guards or janitors at the Titan Wheels factory. Jim worked an eight-hour shift after school, sweeping floors and scrubbing toilets.

At sixteen, Jim dropped out of high school and, with his dad's help, created a stand-up comedy routine. He made his debut at the Yuk Yuk Comedy Club dressed in a mom-made yellow polyester suit with tails. His performance was a disaster. Not discouraged, Jim went on to become a hit at various clubs in the Toronto area.

At eighteen, Jim moved to Los Angeles with a big dream and a thin wallet. He quickly won a regular slot as a stand-up comedian at the Comedy Store. In addition, Jim became the star of the TV series *The Duck Factory*. He was making good money, so he moved his parents from Toronto to his home in L.A.

The good times didn't last. *The Duck Factory* was canceled after only thirteen episodes. Jim was forced to send his parents back to Canada. Despite his difficult situation, Jim's big dream remained intact. One day, he drove up to Mulholland Drive in his rusty old Toyota and looked down over Hollywood. He visualized himself as a massive film star. Then, on a notecard, he drew a check for $10 million made out to himself and post-dated it for Thanksgiving Day, 1995. He folded the check, put it in his wallet, and always carried it with him. Only three days before his father's death, Jim was offered $10 million for the movie *The Mask 2*. He slipped the original notecard into his dad's breast pocket just before they closed the coffin.

Jim Carrey dreams big and lives large. The movies *Ace Ventura, The Mask, Dumb & Dumber, Batman Forever, Liar Liar, The Truman Show, How the Grinch Stole Christmas*, and *Bruce Almighty* are testaments to his big dream, talent, and perseverance.

Big Dreams Are Magical

Big dreams are magical. They accomplish four vital outcomes:

1. *Big dreams put you on the right path.* Big dreams get you off the bench of life and onto the path leading to your big dream. It's vital to be on the right path because harder, faster, and more down the wrong path gets you to where you really don't want to go quicker.

2. *Big dreams put you on a path with other dreamers.* The achievement of your dream will complement the achievement of your fellow travelers' dreams. You will bump into

them occasionally. Now you can work together. People are naturally attracted to big dreamers. Have you ever noticed the dentists who are actively building the practices of their dreams attract the best team members and the best clients?

3. *Big dreams bring you face-to-face with new opportunities.* As you travel down your chosen path, you will see other paths that branch off. Some of these paths will lead you to your dream quicker and more reliably than the one you initially chose. You never would have encountered the new path if you had stayed sitting on the bench of life.

4. *Big dreams are catalysts that mobilize the resources for their achievement.* We often talk to dentists who have dreams for their practices, but they don't take action because they don't have the monetary or skill resources to achieve them. Neither did the U.S. when President John F. Kennedy proclaimed his dream to put a man on the moon and bring him back before the end of the decade. In 1961 the U.S. didn't have the materials or the technical know-how to accomplish a big dream like that. But what did we discover on the way to the dream?—the materials and technology. Like alchemy, the iron was turned into gold. The dream was turned into the reality.

Mental Creation Precedes Physical Creation

Is it just us, or is there something eerily enchanting about the Samuel Taylor Coleridge poem at the beginning of this chapter? There was no flower in your hand at the beginning of the poem. At the end, there was. How could that happen in twelve short lines? And is there a profound message for all of us to learn? We think so.

In the first four lines Coleridge wrote,

"What if you slept?

And what if,

in your sleep

you dreamed?"

You must dream first!

In the next five lines Coleridge wrote,

"And what if,

in your dream,

you went to heaven

and there plucked

a strange and beautiful flower?"

Then, you must mentally possess your dream!

"And what if,

when you awoke,

you had the flower in your hand?"

Now, you will physically possess your dream!

Oprah Winfrey knows about mental creation preceding physical creation. When Oprah started her talk show in Chicago in 1986, she had the big dream of being #1 in the local market. This would be a huge accomplishment with Phil Donohue as competition. Not only did she pass Phil, she went on to create the #1 talk show in the world, a television production company, a wildly successful magazine, and a movie production company.

John F. Kennedy realized that mental creation precedes physical creation. Kennedy's 1961 mental creation of a man on the moon and his ability to sell that creation to a nation led to the physical creation of Neil Armstrong's "One small step for man; one giant leap for mankind."

Get Off Your DOFF

As you move toward your big dream, you may experience one or more of the following emotions:

> Disappointment
>
> Overload
>
> Fear
>
> Frustration

Remember, these emotions aren't bad. They serve a purpose. They're signals that remind you to think or do differently. Here are the four negative emotions and the purposes they serve.

1. *Disappointment* is telling you to keep moving or to change your plan. Success is often just on the other side of the hill from disappointment.

2. *Overload* is telling you to prioritize what's most important in your life and do the most important things first. Or it may be telling you that you need to break a huge task into smaller ones.

3. *Fear* may be telling you to avoid a reality that will physically hurt you. More often, fear is signaling you to do something you've never done before. If this is the case, you need to feel the fear and take action anyway.

4. *Frustration* is telling you to change your approach or to revise your timeline. While writing this book, we felt frus-

trated on several occasions. Then we realized the emotion was our signal to dig into the subject we were frustrated about. Instead of remaining stuck in our frustration, we turned the frustration into fascination and made important new discoveries.

Stop reading this chapter now unless you firmly hold Empowering Belief #9:

I dream big in everything I do.

If you don't have Empowering Belief #9 firmly planted in your mind, the following information will be absolutely useless to you because the actions presented won't match your beliefs.

If you don't hold Empowering Belief #9 and choose to change it now, return to the chapter on How to Change Your Beliefs and follow the instructions.

If you do believe "I dream big in everything I do," read on.

Actions That Exemplify and Reinforce Empowering Belief #9

Here are two important actions that exemplify Empowering Belief #9: I dream big in everything I do.

1. What is the big dream for your practice and your life? Write it in a notebook that will become your Big Dream Journal. Let the dream percolate in your mind for a day or so. Then, go back and revise it.

2. In the past, which of the DOFF emotions have held you back? How will you evaluate them differently this time?

Conclusion

Don't worry about the plan to achieve your dream yet. Take a hint from Dr. Martin Luther King's proclamation, "I have a dream!" He didn't say, "I have a strategic plan." Dr. King knew the "dream" needed to come first. The plan would come later.

13

Empowering Belief #10:
It's an Honor to Be a Dentist

We're honored to be involved in our wonderful profession and to be given the privilege to provide care for those who seek it. Dentistry is one of the few occupations where you can get within inches of people's faces, invade their personal space, and provide treatment at the same time. There are personal friendships where the individuals don't get that close.

It's an Honor to Serve Patients

Our profession isn't just about fixing teeth and healing gums anymore. It's about using the power of close relationships as a vehicle to change people's lives. Our patients become our friends who willingly accept the care we offer. The care enhances their lives, which takes the friendship to a whole new level. We both have hundreds of patients who absolutely love us, and we absolutely love them. We have a purpose that transcends ourselves. We're life changers. That's a whole lot different than being a tooth fixer.

The tag line on most of Matt's ads is *Change Your Smile. Change Your Life.*® Something truly magical happens when people have their smiles improved. Never in a million years did we imagine the power we hold as cosmetic dentists would be so strong. We boost confidence, improve attitudes, and dramatically enhance people's futures.

> "It is one of the beautiful compensations of this life that no one can sincerely try to help another without helping himself."
>
> **—Ralph Waldo Emerson**

But here's the real kicker. In changing hundreds of other people's lives, our lives have been changed, too. We love working 120 days a year so we can be with our families more. We love the financial advantages we possess. We love our profession. If we're not in love with dentistry, our teams and patients won't be either.

It's an Honor to Serve Other Dentists

It's one thing to enhance people's lives with the dentistry we've done. It's a whole new level to help other dentists do the same. We thoroughly enjoy being instructors for the clinical programs at LVI. In addition, we've had thousands of people attend our *Achieving Extreme Success* seminars since 2003. Our purpose in doing the seminars is "to awaken, enliven, and inspire individuals to believe in themselves and to create opportunities for growth, wealth, and abundance through our teachings and talents."

The correspondence we've received from doctors after the program confirms we've done a pretty good job living our purpose. Here's an example:

Thank you for your infectious passion!!! My team is on fire guys. Two full mouths at 38k each on credit card since our return on Tuesday!!! We also had a gal book her 26k treatment today as well!!! What a kick ass class; and you have made it much easier to have fun and take the 'doctor' image bullshit out of the way. No tie since return and feelin great. We prepped a full mouth (upper) yesterday and had energy and laughter throughout the day. You both rock! I love your approach to life and our profession.

Dr. Rod Spencer, Val, Michele, Kim and Sally

An Honor and an Opportunity to Give Back

We believe it's an honor to be dentists. We're two of a select group of people who have been given the privilege to practice dentistry. That's a big deal to us. We also realize that with every honor comes an opportunity to give back.

We give the highest quality dentistry available to our patients. In our minds, not providing the best care (the kind you would give your loved ones) to people is the equivalent of ethical malpractice. *They* may not know what the best care is, but we can guarantee your gut knows. You can cover up the gut feeling with denial or other potions, but it's always there, constantly eating away at you.

It's not worth it! Life is too short. Today you need to make the commitment to head down the path to practice excellence. During the process, you need to intelligently power through the real and imagined barriers that have been holding you back. You need to make the choice to be the best dentist in the area.

Even though we always provide the highest *quality* dentistry to our patients, we can't always provide the optimal *quantity*. Sometimes people can't afford or don't want to have all their dentistry completed right away. We understand that. We're not "all-or-nothing" dentists. But we always give people a shot at comprehensive restorative and cosmetic dentistry. Many of them decide to do it. They love the results and refer their family and friends. And all the while our practices keep rolling along.

We also have an opportunity to provide dentistry to deserving people who can't afford it. As we've said before, we feel it's important that we choose them, not that they choose us. Finally, we have an opportunity to help others learn what we know.

There are various ways to give back. Assuming you feel it's an honor to be a dentist, the way you choose depends on your unique purpose in life and the values you hold dear.

> "Life is a gift, and it offers each of us the privilege, the opportunity and the responsibility to give something back by becoming more."
>
> **—Anthony Robbins**

The Last at Bat

We're sure Babe Ruth felt honored to be a baseball legend and a role model to millions. Babe spent his final days at the Sloan-Kettering Cancer Center in New York City. One morning a nurse found him standing on an outside balcony, watching a group of young boys playing baseball.

"Watch the swing on that kid," Ruth said with admiration. "Go down there and tell that kid to step into the plate and lean forward on his swing. He could be a real good hitter."

The nurse did as requested, pointing out to the boy he had a mentor. The boys gave Ruth, high on his hospital balcony, a wave.

The next day, Ruth summoned the nurse again. "I want you to give that kid this bat for me," he said weakly, holding out one he had signed.

Babe Ruth gave back to the very end. He died later that evening.

> **Stop reading this chapter now unless you firmly hold Empowering Belief #10:**
>
> **It's an honor to be a dentist.**
>
> If you don't have Empowering Belief #10 firmly planted in your mind, the following information will be absolutely useless to you because the actions presented won't match your beliefs.
>
> If you don't hold Empowering Belief #10 and choose to change it now, return to the chapter on How to Change Your Beliefs and follow the instructions.
>
> If you do believe that "it's an honor to be a dentist," read on.

Actions That Exemplify and Reinforce Empowering Belief #10

Here are three actions that exemplify Empowering Belief #10: It's an honor to be a dentist.

1. What's your purpose as a dentist? Write your answer in your Big Dream Journal. If you have trouble answering the question, ask yourself these follow-up questions:

- What's truly important to you?
- What are you all about, really?
- Why do you come to work every day?
- What good are you in the world?
- What do you stand for?

> "This is the true joy in life, to be used for a purpose recognized by yourself as a mighty one.
>
> Being thoroughly used up and worn out before you are thrown on the scrap heap.
>
> Being a force of nature instead of a feverish, selfish, little clod of ailments and grievances complaining that the world will not devote itself to making you happy."
>
> **—George Bernard Shaw**

2. What quality dentistry do you give back to your patients? If it's not the best, what's your plan to make it so?

3. In what ways do you give back to the people in your area? What is your plan to give more?

Conclusion

This is the last of the ten empowering beliefs that return like boomerangs to create our success in dentistry and life. When studying people's lives, it's natural to look at what they have (the end of the boomerang's flight). We believe it's more important to examine what they believe (the beginning of the flight). See, *it all begins with you and the beliefs you choose to hold!* When you really get that last sentence, your entire life will change for the better. You will stop complaining about all the external people, events, and situations you think are controlling your life and start focusing on your internal thoughts, emotions, and the actions they promote. You will stop feeling helpless and hopeless and start feeling empowered and emboldened. You will stop just making a living and start designing a life.

Section 3

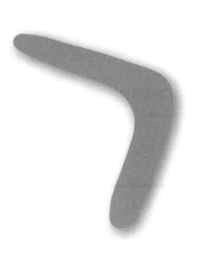

Harmonic Wealth®

A vocal group is composed of two or more individual singers. Each singer has a unique voice and sings a specific part of the total musical score. The vocal group is in harmony when everybody sings their parts well and blends with the other singers.

Likewise, your overall wealth is composed of five different areas. The term Harmonic Wealth® was coined by James Arthur Ray. Harmonic Wealth is created when each of the five areas of your life is healthy and in harmony with the other four areas. The five areas of Harmonic Wealth are:

1. *relational*: your family, business, and community relationships
2. *mental/emotional*: your thoughts, beliefs, and the emotions they produce
3. *spiritual*: your connection with the Universal Power
4. *physical*: your health and vitality
5. *financial*: your income, expense balance, and savings plan

This section has two chapters. In the first chapter, you will set goals in one or more of the five Harmonic Wealth areas. In the second chapter, you will discover how to create the future you deserve.

So let's get started. The auditorium is full, and the curtain is rising. It's show time.

14

Setting SMART Goals

Back in the Empowering Belief #9 chapter, you identified your big dream and wrote it in your Big Dream Journal. In this chapter, you're going to create goals in one or more of the five areas of Harmonic Wealth. Each of the goals will be a stepping stone that creates the path to your big dream.

SMART Goals

In his book *Make Success Measurable*, Douglas K. Smith used SMART as an acronym for the five characteristics he believed all goals should have. We have modified his concepts a little in this chapter. To us, a SMART goal is:

> **S**pecific
>
> **M**easurable
>
> **A**ccountable
>
> **R**ealistic
>
> **T**imed

Specific

A SMART goal is specific. You should know precisely what the goal is. "I'm going to work out" is a non-specific goal. "I'm going to the twenty-four-hour fitness facility on Monday, Tuesday, Thursday, and Friday next week at 3 P.M. and do seventy-five minutes of stretching, resistance work and aerobic exercise" is a specific goal.

Measurable

A SMART goal is measurable. Each goal should have a number(s) attached to it so you know the goal has been achieved. "Go for a walk" is a non-measurable goal. "Go for a two-mile walk in thirty minutes" is measurable.

Accountable

A SMART goal is accountable. When setting a goal, you need to be fully accountable for its achievement. You can't control the behavior of others, so their actions can't be factored into the successful achievement of your goal.

An example of a non-accountable goal would be to have a romantic relationship with a specific person in seven days. You can't control what the other person does. You can only control what you do. So the goal should be changed to something like, "By the end of the week, I will ask Maria to go on a date."

Here's another example of a non-accountable goal. "I will win the lottery within a year." You can't control how ping pong balls fall out of a machine no matter how hard you try. A better, accountable goal would be to put $3,000 into your retirement account every month for the next year.

Realistic

A SMART goal is realistic. As we mentioned earlier in this book, be careful how you use the word "realistic." Sometimes, people limit themselves when they say, "It's not realistic." To be realistic, your goal must be something you believe you can achieve. If you set a goal you think might be unachievable, your doubt will be planted into your unconscious mind and hinder your actions and results.

Whatever you firmly believe you can achieve, no matter how large it seems to others, is a realistic goal for you. You're currently using a fraction of the unlimited potential you have inside. Set your goals high. Most importantly, believe you will achieve. We have never for a moment doubted our ability to build the practices of our dreams. Our unquestioned belief was the spark that ignited us to take the actions that led to success.

Timed

A SMART goal is timed. Each outcome goal should have a precise time limit for its attainment. Some goals are outcome goals and some are process goals. "Climbing a fourteen thousand-foot peak by August 1, 2010" is an outcome goal with a time limit for its achievement. "Going to the twenty-four-hour fitness facility on Monday, Tuesday, Thursday, and Friday next week at 3 P.M. and doing seventy-five minutes of stretching, resistance work and aerobic exercise" is a weekly process goal. Process goals have beginning and ending times.

Harmonic Wealth® Smart Goals

In the introduction to this section, you learned that it's important to be wealthy in five areas of your life. The five areas of Harmonic Wealth are:

1. *relational*: your family, business, and community relationships

2. *mental*: your thoughts, beliefs, and the emotions they produce

3. *spiritual*: your connection with the Universal Power

4. *physical*: your health and vitality

5. *financial*: your income, expense balance, and savings plan

In this chapter, you will set a series of SMART goals in one or more of the Harmonic Wealth areas. Don't overdo this at first. If you wanted to make your bicep muscles stronger, you would start with lighter weights and fewer repetitions. As you got stronger, you would add weights and do more reps.

It's the same with achieving goals. Pick a few short-term goals that are especially important to you. Make sure they're attainable. After you attain the goals, set longer-term goals and expand your goals to more areas of your life.

> "Have confidence that if you do a small thing well, you can do a bigger thing well, too."
>
> **—Joseph Story**

Relational Goals

Tony Robbins said, "The quality of your life is the quality of your relationships." We agree. That's why you may want to start your goal-setting exercise with relational goals. Pick one important family relationship you have and write it in your Big Dream Journal. Then set a one-day goal for that relationship.

We like one-day goals. They usually involve doing a small thing—and by doing the small thing you gain momentum needed to do bigger things. Here's an example of a one-day family relationship goal. "Tomorrow, I'm going to tell Mary I love her three times—once in the morning as I leave for work, once when we first meet after work, and once right before we go to bed."

After you achieve the one-day goal, set a one-week goal and write it in your Big Dream Journal. For example: "For the next seven days, I'm going to give Mary a big hug and tell her I love her at least three times a day." After you achieve that weekly process goal, you can move on to an additional one-month

outcome goal. For example: "For the next thirty days, I'm going to give Mary a big hug and tell her I love her at least three
times a day. In addition, we're going together on a surprise,
three-day get-away to Santa Barbara before May 15th."

After you've strengthened your personal relationship
muscle, you can move to one of your business relationships.
Pick an important relationship and set a series of SMART goals.
Make sure there is a 95 percent chance the goal will be at-
tained. Success breeds success.

Mental Goals

Mental goals can be intellectual or emotional in nature.
Here's an example of an emotional goal: Let's say you want to
experience the emotion of happiness more consistently. Make
your daily goal to form happiness-producing thoughts five times
a day. In addition, whenever you feel unhappy, notice what
thought is producing the emotion and immediately change it.
Finally, you can do a happiness-producing activity for thirty
minutes.

After you've done that, you can move to a longer time-
span goal for the same emotion and add another emotion.

An example of a one-day intellectual goal would be to read
an inspiring biography or autobiography for thirty minutes.

Spiritual Goals

In your Big Dream Journal, create a one-day spiritual goal
for an action you're committed to taking to improve your connection with the Universal Power.

Here's an example of a one-day spiritual goal. "Tomorrow,
I'm committed to meditating twenty minutes in the morning
and twenty minutes in the evening." After you've done that,
you will want to extend that goal and perhaps add an addi-

tional goal of going on a five-day spiritual retreat within the next four months.

Physical Goals

When the time is right, set a one-day goal you're committed to taking to improve your physical well-being. Then set a weekly goal. An example of a weekly process goal would be to go to the gym four days in the next week to do seventy-five minutes of stretching, resistance training, and aerobic exercise. A monthly outcome goal may be to lose two pounds of fat by a combination of the weekly exercise previously mentioned and drinking a protein shake in the afternoon and only eating a piece of fresh fruit in the evening.

Financial Goals

When the time is right, in your Big Dream Journal, set a one-day goal you're committed to taking to improve your financial situation. The one-day goal could be to sign up for a savings plan at work in which 10 percent of every paycheck is automatically deposited to your retirement account. A one-month goal could be to gross $60,000 in your dental practice.

Approach Your Goals with Confidence

Confidence is the positive expectation of a favorable outcome. In other words, confidence is a belief system. Confidence must be experienced in appropriate doses. Over-confidence leads to cockiness. Under-confidence is just as bad, because it leads to cowardice.

Confidence is the fuel that fires the self-fulfilling prophecy phenomenon. Your life is a continual series of "now" moments. Each "now" affects all future "now" moments. If you feel confident that some event will occur, you increase the likelihood of it coming to pass through a self-fulfilling prophecy. The opposite is also true. So your success in life or in business isn't a single event. It's a long-term chain of confident "now" moments strung together from the present moment to the attainment of your big dream.

Conclusion

The greatest basketball player to play the game is Michael Jordan. He knows a thing or two about confidence. Jordan has said, "You have to expect things of yourself before you can do them." In this chapter, you set SMART goals in five different areas of your life. In effect, you made it very clear what you expect from yourself. Now you need to do them. That's the subject of our next chapter. Keep reading. There are twelve seconds left on the clock, and twenty thousand people are counting on you to confidently make the last shot.

15

Creating the Future You Deserve

The big dream you've created is the vision in the distance you're moving toward. The SMART goals you set in the last chapter are the mileage markers along the path. They break the journey into smaller segments and then give you reinforcement as you pass them. As you move down your road less traveled, you will want to be enthusiastic and intelligent.

Be Enthusiastic

Muhammad Ali said, "Champions aren't made in the gyms. Champions are made from something they have deeper inside them—a desire, a dream, a vision. They have last-minute stamina. They have to be a little faster. They have to have the skill and the will. But the will must be stronger than the skill."

"The will must be stronger than the skill." How true. We occasionally see dentists wanting to transform their practices. They have all the necessary skills to do so. But they don't have the will to propel themselves through the challenging times that will invariably pop up.

So where does will come from? We believe it's the combination of a firm belief in the achievement of a big dream and acting enthusiastically in the pursuit of that dream. The word "enthusiasm" is derived from the Greek word *éntheos* meaning "possessed by a god" or "inspired." That's a hint!

There are two ways you can generate enthusiasm—mentally and physically. The best way to generate enthusiasm mentally is to feel enthusiastic and identify what you were thinking about or focusing on to feel that way. Vividly imagining living your dream with all five senses is always an effective way to feel enthusiastic.

To generate enthusiasm physically, act *as if* you were living your dream now. Move your body the way that person would. Put the same expression on your face that person would have. Talk in the same way that person would talk. Your movements will send goal-achieving messages to your brain, to the Universal Power, and to other people. With time, you will become the person you pretend to be.

"We are what we pretend to be.
So we must be careful what we pretend to be."

—Kurt Vonnegut

Be Intelligent

People who are just excited but don't know what they're doing are dangerous. We don't want you to be dangerous. We want you to be intelligent. Here are nine ways:

1. Start your big dream journey from where you're at right now. Don't wait for something to happen before you begin. Every journey begins with the first step—and it's often the most difficult one to take.

2. Learn from other people's experience. Don't recreate the wheel. Read books. Attend seminars. Get a mentor.

3. Get a knowledgeable and caring coach to help you with the skills needed for the journey. Tiger Woods is by far the

best golfer playing today, and he still has a coach who consistently gives him valuable feedback.

4. On your journey, remember what's truly important in life. Take great care of the people you love along the way.

5. Take excellent care of yourself. If you "blow a tire," your journey will come to a screeching halt.

6. Sharpen your axe every once in a while by consistently learning new skills. You will cut down more trees at the end of the day.

7. Create an intelligent and personalized action plan to get you from where you are now to where you want to go.

8. Think evolution not revolution. *Do not* look at our practices and attempt to do the same thing in six months. *Do* move toward your dream practice one step at a time. Some steps you will be able to take quickly. Some take more time.

9. Help others achieve their dreams. Start with your family and dental team members.

Criticism and Resistance

We both ran into some harsh criticism and formidable obstacles on the paths to our dream practices. So will you. When some bench-sitter criticizes you, remember this question: "If someone offers you a gift, and you don't accept the gift, to whom does the gift belong?" It certainly doesn't belong to you. It belongs to the other person. So, when someone offers you criticism, don't accept it (unless you believe it's valid).

You're also going to meet resistance. Resistance is terribly misunderstood. Most people think resistance holds them back. On the contrary, when used correctly resistance helps you progress toward your dream. The air resistance in an eagle's face is the same stuff the eagle pushes against to move forward. The air resistance in the eagle's face is the same material that flows over its wings to provide lift. The air resistance is a necessity for flight. If the air resistance were gone, the eagle would be in a vacuum and fall to the ground.

Six Ways to Talk Yourself Out of Taking Action

This is the last chapter of the book. Very soon, you're going to have to make a decision to apply the information you've learned. Many dentists are great at talking themselves out of taking action—even if the action will improve their practices and lives. Check out the following six ways. If you're thinking any of them right now, follow our advice.

1. *You believe you can't do it.* If you believe this one, take the $1 million test. If I gave you $1 million to do the thing you believe you can't do, would you do it? If your answer is "yes," you *can* do it.

2. *You try to do it.* There is no such thing as "try." You either do something or you don't do something. Decide which it's going to be and get on with your life.

3. *You don't think you have enough time.* You've got all the time there is. If time were money, you would be a multi-billionaire. How much TV do you watch each week? You have time for that.

4. *You procrastinate.* You say, "I'll do it tomorrow" or "Someday I'll do it." To overcome procrastination, do the following:

   a. Make binding commitments to other people.
   b. Break large tasks into small parts and do one part at a time.

    c. Take the rocking chair test. Imagine how you are going to feel sitting in a rocking chair at the old-folks home knowing that you didn't begin the journey to your dream.

    d. Reconnect with achieving your dream. How are you going to feel when you live your dream?

5. *You have a bad case of the terrible "toos."* You say to yourself, "I'm too old," "I'm too tired," I'm too poor," "It will take too much time." Baloney! Colonel Sanders wasn't too old to start his Kentucky Fried Chicken franchise operation. He was sixty-five! Oprah Winfrey wasn't too poor to begin her journey to being one of the richest and most powerful women in America. She had almost no financial assets when she began her local talk show in Chicago. Today she has a net worth of $2.5 billion.

6. *You believe that you need to be an expert before you begin your journey.* Remember, the resources needed will come to you if you have a big dream and if you keep moving down the path.

Conclusion

In the I Dream Big in Everything I Do chapter, you read about President Kennedy's dream to put a man on the moon before the end of the decade. Kennedy's dream came true on July 20, 1969. The movie *Apollo 13* opens with a gathering of astronauts at the home of Jim and Marilyn Lovell on that special day. The people are there to watch a live television broadcast of their fellow astronaut, Neil Armstrong, setting foot on the moon. As veteran newsman Walter Cronkite describes the event, we hear Armstrong utter his famous words, "One small step for man; one giant leap for mankind." The group becomes strangely quiet, joining Cronkite in being overwhelmed by the significance of the moment.

After the broadcast is over, the party breaks up, and everyone goes home. The Tom Hanks character, Jim Lovell, is now alone with his wife Marilyn in their backyard. Looking up at the moon, Lovell says, "From now on, we live in a world where man has walked on the moon. It's not a miracle. *We just decided to go.*"

"We just decided to go." Simple words with a profound message. Deciding to go is the most important step on the journey to the practice and life of your dreams. Unfortunately, it's usually the step not taken. Most dentists never decide to go. They never decide to create the practice of their dreams. They may think about it, talk about it, attend programs that teach how to do it, and write lofty mission statements that proclaim it. But they never decide to go.

The word "decide" is derived from the Latin word "*decidere,*" meaning "to cut off." When you decide to do something, you literally cut off the possibility of not doing it. You never allow failure to enter the equation. You burn your bridges behind you. There is no turning back as you head down the path. You keep putting one foot ahead of the other as you march through rugged terrain and bad weather. When you fall down, you get up. When people try to discourage you or put obstacles in your way, you pay no attention to them and climb over the barriers. When you come to a fork in the path, you choose the road less traveled by. You are not denied…no matter what.

And slowly but surely you arrive at the practice and life of your dreams. You look around and smile. It isn't a miracle. You just decided to go.

Authors' Products and Services

Achieving Extreme Success Seminar

Achieving Extreme Success is an energetic and highly motivating two-day seminar where you will discover the success secrets of extremely successful dental practices from the people who are doing it.

In *Achieving Extreme Success*, you will learn:

- why most dental practices struggle while a few consistently have record-breaking years
- how to market your practice effectively to attract people who desire the kinds of care you want to deliver
- how to create practice separation from the other offices in your area
- how to communicate with people so they ask you to do their comprehensive dentistry
- why most dentists are stuck doing single-tooth, insurance-dictated dentistry while a few are routinely performing comprehensive aesthetic and reconstructive dentistry
- how to create a High-Octane Team of people who work together and do their best work
- how to produce Harmonic Wealth® in all areas of your life

Achieving Extreme Success is inspirational and practical. Your team and you will leave fired-up to use the practical skills that transform good dental practices into great ones! Learn more at www.BynumMoweryWay.com.

Achieving Extreme Success In-Office Coaching

Bring a Bynum Mowery Way trained coach into your office to help you implement the Achieving Extreme Success principles in your practice. Go to www.BynumMoweryWay.com for details.

Achieving Extreme Success Phone Coaching

Speak with a Bynum Mowery Way trained coach on the phone to help you create and implement an Achieving Extreme Success plan of action in your office. Visit www.BynumMoweryWay.com for details.

Achieving Extreme Success Products

Check out our ever-expanding collection of Achieving Extreme Success CD and DVD products at www.BynumMowery Way.com.

AUTHOR RECOMMENDED PRODUCTS AND SERVICES

Las Vegas Institute for Advanced Dental Studies

To learn more about the Las Vegas Institute for Advanced Dental Studies and its programs, go to www.lviglobal.com or call 702-341-7978.

Las Vegas Institute for Advanced Dental Studies
9501 Hillwood Drive
Las Vegas, NV 89134

James Arthur Ray

To learn more about James Arthur Ray and his programs, go to www.jamesray.com or call 760-476-9077.

James Ray International
5927 Balfour Court, Ste 104
Carlsbad, CA 92008

Aurum Ceramic Dental Laboratory

We choose Aurum Ceramic Laboratory to do all our restorations. If you want to be the best dentist and do the best dentistry, you need to use the best laboratory. There is nobody better than Aurum.

Aurum Ceramic Dental Laboratory
www.aurumgroup.com
800-363-3989

Nate Booth Products and Services

Check out all of Nate Booth's books, audio/video training programs, in-office and phone coaching programs and presentations for dental groups at www.natebooth.com.

Nate Booth & Associates
www.natebooth.com
800-917-0008

Give the Gift of

The Boomerang Effect
for Dental Professionals

How Your Beliefs Return to Create
Your Personal and Professional Lives

USE THIS FORM OR ORDER ONLINE

❑ **YES**, I want _____ copies of *The Boomerang Effect for Dental Professionals* at $69.95 each, plus $4.95 shipping per book (South Carolina residents please add $4.20 sales tax per book). Canadian orders must be accompanied by a postal money order in U.S. funds. Allow 15 days for delivery.

❑ **YES**, I am interested in having Dr. Matt Bynum or Dr. Art Mowery give a presentation to my company or an association to which I belong. Please send information.

My check or money order for $_____ is enclosed.

Please charge my: ❑ Visa   ❑ MasterCard
                   ❑ Discover ❑ American Express

Name _____

Organization _____

Address _____

City/State/Zip _____

Phone_____ Email_____

Card # _____

Exp. Date_____ Signature _____

Please make your check payable and return to:

Hakalau Publishing Company
1334 S. Hwy. 14, Simpsonville, SC 29681

Call your credit card order to: 864-297-5585
Fax: 864-297-4166

Or order online at: BynumMoweryWay.com